妇科学聚焦

Gynaecology

IN*focus*

注　意

医学在不断进步。虽然有关安全问题的注意事项必须遵守，但是由于新的研究和临床经验在不断拓宽我们的知识，在治疗和用药方面做出某些改变也许是必需或适宜的。建议读者核对所开每种药品生产厂商的最新产品信息，确认推荐剂量、服药方法、时间和禁忌证。决定患者服药剂量和最佳治疗方式的责任在于实施治疗的医师，即有赖于其个人经验和对每位患者的了解而定。出版商和著者对可能引起的人身或财产的任何损伤和（或）损失，不承担任何责任。

出版者

妇科学聚焦

Gynaecology IN *focus*

原　著　Janice Rymer
Andrew N J Fish

主　译　郑建华　黄明莉

译　者（以姓氏笔画为序）
尤　琪　刘运铎　曲晓力
郑建华　贲　崴　黄可金
黄明莉　彭春杰

北京大学医学出版社
Peking University Medical Press

Gynaecology in Focus
Janice Rymer, Andrew Fish
ISBN-13: 978-0-443-07437-0
ISBN-10: 0-443-07437-2

Authorized Simplified Chinese translation from English language edition published by the Proprietor.
978-981-259-561-4
981-259-561-9

Elsevier (Singapore) Pte Ltd.
3 Killiney Road, #08-01 Winsland House I, Singapore 239519
Tel: (65) 6349-0200, Fax: (65) 6733-1817
First Published 2007
2007 年初版

北京市版权局著作权合同登记号：图字：01-2006-1817

图书在版编目（CIP）数据

妇科学聚焦：英汉对照 /（英）赖默（Rymer，J.），（英）菲什（Fish，A.）著；郑建华，黄明莉译. —北京：北京大学医学出版社，2007.9

书名原文：Gynaecology in Focus

ISBN 978-7-81071-985-8

I. 妇… II. ①赖… ②菲… ③郑… ④黄… III. 妇科学—英、汉 IV. R711

中国版本图书馆 CIP 数据核字（2007）第 106426 号

妇科学聚焦

主　　译：郑建华　黄明莉
出版发行：北京大学医学出版社 (电话：010-82802230)
地　　址：(100083) 北京市海淀区学院路 38 号　北京大学医学部院内
网　　址：http://www.pumpress.com.cn
E-mail：booksale@bjmu.edu.cn
印　　刷：莱芜市圣龙印务有限责任公司
经　　销：新华书店
责任编辑：刘　燕　　责任校对：杜　悦　　责任印制：郭桂兰
开　　本：889mm × 1194mm　1/32　印张：8.75　字数：279 千字
版　　次：2008 年 1 月第 1 版　2008 年 1 月第 1 次印刷
书　　号：ISBN 978-7-81071-985-8
定　　价：63.00 元

译者前言

《妇科学聚焦》一书包含了大量的临床图片，行文简洁流畅，易懂易记，具有很高的实用性。各章节篇幅不长，虽无深奥理论，但重点突出，概念清晰准确，诊疗方法翔实，包括了妇科领域最新进展，有助于提高妇科医师的诊疗水平。

本书是英汉对照版本，在获得医学知识的同时还可以提高专业英语水平，既可供医学生、研究生、住院医师、全科医师学习和提高，也可作为专科医生参考借鉴之用。

在翻译此书的过程中我们尽量做到词准意达，但是由于水平有限，可能存在不足之处，请各位同仁赐教指正。

郑建华

2007 年 6 月

于哈尔滨医科大学第一附属医院

致　谢

我们非常感谢为这本图书提供一些图片的人员: John Dewhurst 先生，R J S Harries 医生，J Robinson 医生，D H Oram 先生，S Thorpe 医生，P Greenhouse 医生，M Hooper 女士，S Barton 医生，R Jelley 医生，R Forman 先生，I Fogelan 教授，C Brown 医生，F Mitchell 医生，A Cutner 先生，C Kelleher 先生，Y Khalaf 先生，J Robinson 女士，J Dent 女士，S Pugh 女士，Royal College of Surgeons，以及 Gower 医学出版社。我们应该尤其感谢 E Lombard 医生、Has Ahmed 先生和 Chapman 教授，他们允许我们使用以前和他们共同出版的书籍中的资料。我们感谢下述医院的图像科: Guy 和 St Thomas 医院，Royal London 医院、Brighton 和 Sussex 大学医院，以及同意拍照的妇女。

目录

Contents

进行妇科诊断

病史

一个完整的病史对于确诊妇科疾病是必要的。

环境

检查的环境应确保私密性，令患者感觉舒适，患者在检查之前不应该被要求脱衣服。

内容

与下列相关的特殊信息应该被采集：

- 产次
- 末次月经
- 月经周期的长短
- 避孕的应用
- 上次宫颈涂片的时间。

应清楚地确定患者当前的主诉，并填写既往妇产科病史（图1）。记录性生活是很重要的：包括目前性关系的持续时间及性伴侣是否有改变。为防止可疑感染，必须询问性伴侣的症状。

检查：体位

对病人行盆腔检查可采取仰卧位或左侧卧位（图2，3）。西姆斯体位（类似于昏迷体位）也可采用。仰卧位便于检查外生殖器，特别是外阴、阴唇、阴蒂及尿道。

1 Making a gynaecological diagnosis

History

A thorough history is essential to make an accurate gynaecological diagnosis.

Setting

The setting for the interview should ensure privacy and comfort for the woman, who should not be asked to undress before being interviewed.

Content

Specific information should be gathered regarding:

- parity
- last menstrual period
- length of the menstrual cycle
- contraceptive use
- date of the last cervical smear.

The presenting complaint should be clearly defined and put in the context of the previous obstetric and gynaecological history (Fig. 1). It is important to record information about sexual activity: duration of the present sexual relationship and any recent change in sexual partner. In cases of suspected infection it is mandatory to ask about the symptoms of the partner(s).

Examination: Positions

A pelvic examination can be performed with the patient either in the dorsal position or in the left lateral position (Figs 2,3). Sims position, which is similar to the coma position, may also be used. In the dorsal position the external genitalia are easily inspected, with particular reference to the vulva, labia, clitoris and urethra.

卫生监督所

姓 先生 / 夫人 / 小姐

单元号

D.O.B.

医院

会诊医师

名

日期	内容	妇科
	年龄　产次　末次月经 –/–/–	
	月经周期 /　避孕方法　上次宫颈涂片时间 –/–/–	
	主诉	
	既往妇产科病史	
	既往医疗史	
	社会史或家族史　药物	
	过敏	
	临床所见	

图 1　病历表
History sheet

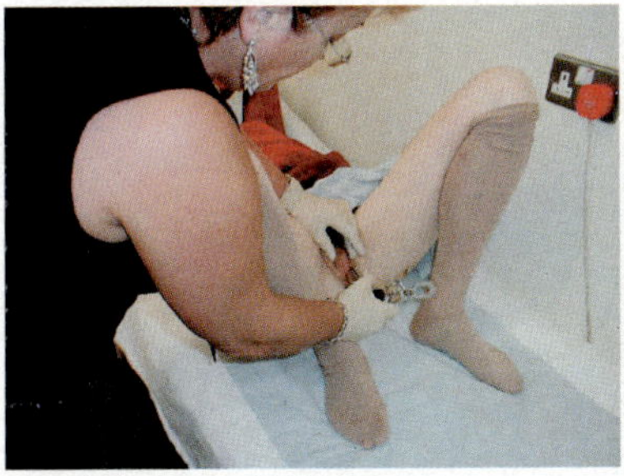

图 2　仰卧位检查
Examination in the dorsal position

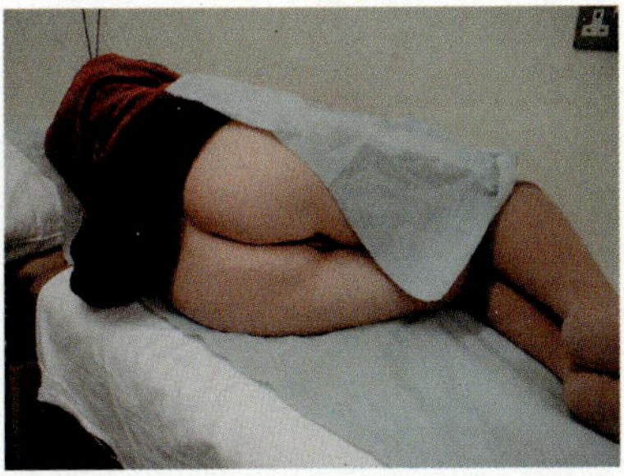

图 3　左侧卧位患者
Patient in the left lateral position

检查：仪器和方法

双瓣窥器

双瓣窥器被用来检查宫颈和阴道壁（图4）。也可用于做宫颈涂片和宫颈内拭子检查。

双合诊检查

进行双合诊检查用来评估盆腔脏器。两手戴上手套。右手一个或两个手指涂上润滑剂，插入阴道内用来抬举并固定子宫和附件，以便于位于腹部上的左手能触摸到盆腔脏器（图5）。确定子宫和附件的大小、位置（前倾、成轴、后倾）、子宫活动度，以及是否伴有压痛和/或穹窿的包块。宫颈刺激症是当检查者的手移动宫颈引起阔韧带拉伸时一侧或另一侧附件触痛。

西姆斯窥器

左侧卧位适用于西姆斯窥器检查（图6）。该窥器最初是设计用来检查膀胱阴道瘘。现在常用来评估子宫阴道脱垂。窥器的一个末端插入阴道内，并轻轻地向后牵拉。由此可以看到阴道的前壁。为了观察阴道后壁，可在缓慢撤下西姆斯窥器的同时向阴道内插入一副海绵夹持钳以使阴道前壁回缩。

Bivalve speculum

A bivalve speculum is used to inspect the cervix and the vaginal walls (Fig. 4). It is also used when taking cervical smears and endocervical swabs.

Bimanual examination

A bimanual examination is performed to assess the pelvic organs. Gloves are used on both hands. One or two lubricated fingers of the right hand are inserted into the vagina and used to elevate and steady the uterus and adnexa so that the left hand on the abdomen can feel the pelvic organs (Fig. 5). The size, position (anteverted, axial or retroverted) and mobility of the uterus are determined together with the presence of tenderness and/or masses in the fornices. *Cervical excitation* is defined as tenderness that arises in one or other adnexum when the broad ligament is stretched by movement of the cervix with the examining fingers.

Sims speculum

The left lateral position facilitates the use of a Sims speculum (Fig. 6). This instrument was originally designed for displaying vesicovaginal fistulae. It is now more often used in the assessment of uterovaginal prolapse. One end of the speculum is inserted into the vagina and gentle traction is applied backwards. The anterior vaginal wall is thus visualized. To view the posterior vaginal wall, a pair of sponge-holding forceps are inserted to retract the anterior vaginal wall while the Sims speculum is slowly withdrawn.

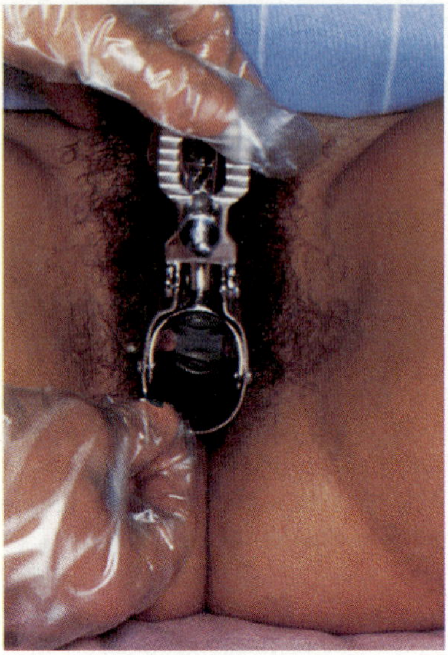

图 4　应用双瓣窥器检查
Examination with a bivalve speculum

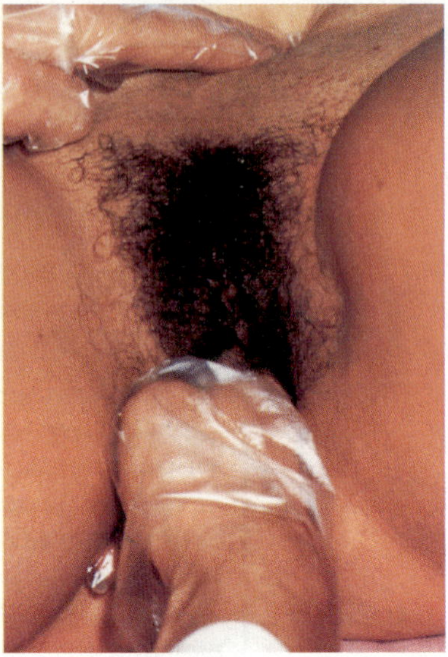

图 5　双合诊检查
Bimanual examination

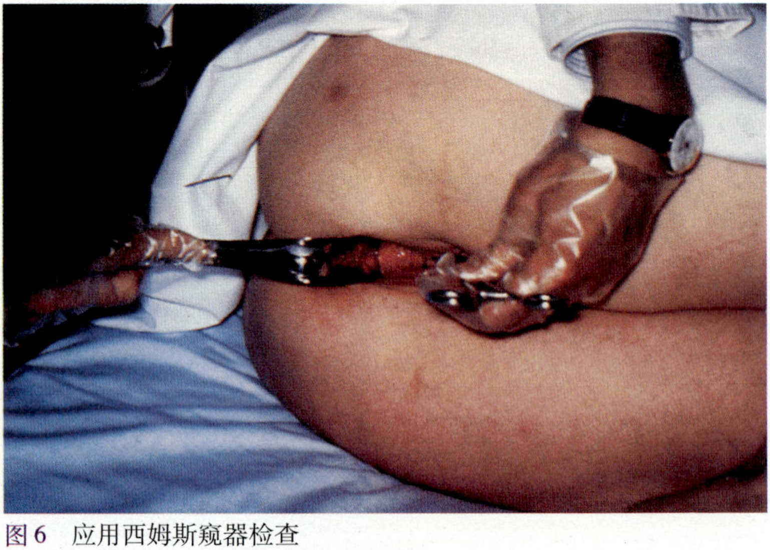

图 6　应用西姆斯窥器检查
Examination using a Sims speculum

进行宫颈涂片

使用双瓣窥器充分暴露宫颈。用木质刮板的窄端插入宫颈管内使其边缘紧靠宫颈（图7)。紧贴宫颈旋转 360° 后移开。刮板上收集的标本在载玻片上均匀铺开后（图8a)，立刻浸入固定液中（3%醋酸溶于 95% 酒精）。

现在正在引进液基细胞学。如图7那样采集标本后在转移液中搅动（图 8b)，使实验室准备的玻片更易于读片。

适应证

所有性生活活跃的妇女应每三年进行一次涂片。英国宫颈筛查计划包括所有20 ~ 65岁妇女，每3 ~ 5年筛查一次。

进行微生物拭子检查

使用双瓣窥器，用高位阴道拭子从阴道后穹窿取材。将棉拭子置于适当的转移液中。

适应证

高位阴道拭子用来检查下生殖道病原体，例如白色念珠菌或阴道滴虫，这些病原体会引起阴道分泌物增多和外阴刺激症状。宫颈内拭子通常用来检查有可能播散至上生殖道并引起盆腔炎疾病的病原体，例如沙眼衣原体和淋球菌。这些微生物可感染柱状上皮。这种微生物拭子应插入宫颈管内（图9）搅动后再撤出，并置于合适的转移液中。

Taking a cervical smear

The cervix should be clearly visualized using a bivalve speculum. The narrow point of the wooden spatula is inserted into the endocervical canal so that the lip rests against the cervix (Fig. 7). It is then rotated through 360° , keeping in firm contact with the cervix, and then removed. The material collected on the spatula is spread evenly on a microscope slide (Fig. 8a) which is immediately immersed in fixative (3% acetic acid in 95% alcohol).

Liquid-based cytology is being introduced. The sample is taken as in Figure 7 and agitated in the transport medium (Fig. 8b) enabling the laboratory to prepare slides that are easier to read.

Indications

All sexually active women should have smears taken at 3-yearly intervals. The National Cervical Screening Programme in the UK includes all women 20~65 years, 3~5-yearly.

Taking microbiological swabs

High vaginal swabs are taken from the posterior fornix using a bivalve speculum. The cotton-tipped swab is placed in the appropriate transport medium.

Indications

High vaginal swabs are used to detect lower genital tract pathogens, e.g. *Candida albicans or Trichomonas vaginalis*, which give rise to symptoms such as discharge and vulval irritation. Endocervical swabs are used to detect pathogens that may spread to the upper genital tract and cause pelvic inflammatory disease, e.g. *Chlamydia trachomatis* and *Neisseria gonorrhoeae*. These bacteria infect columnar epithelium. The microbiological swab should be inserted into the endocervical canal (Fig. 9), agitated and withdrawn. It should then be placed in the appropriate transport medium.

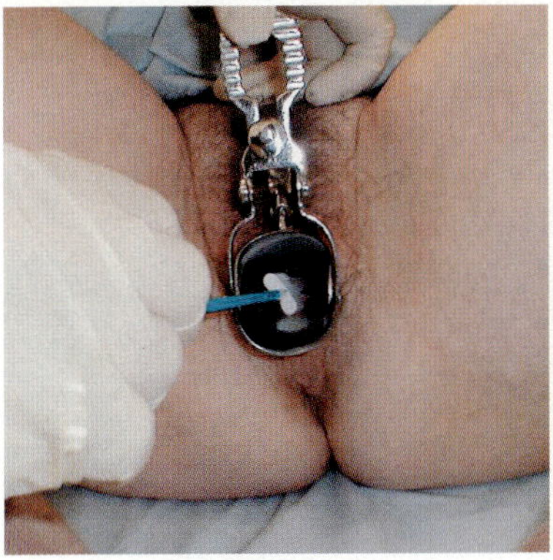

图 7 进行宫颈涂片
Taking a cervical smear

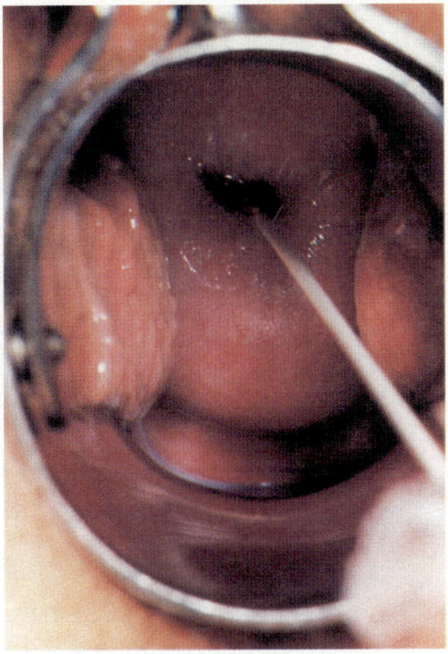

图 9 进行宫颈管拭子检查
Taking an endocervical swab

a.

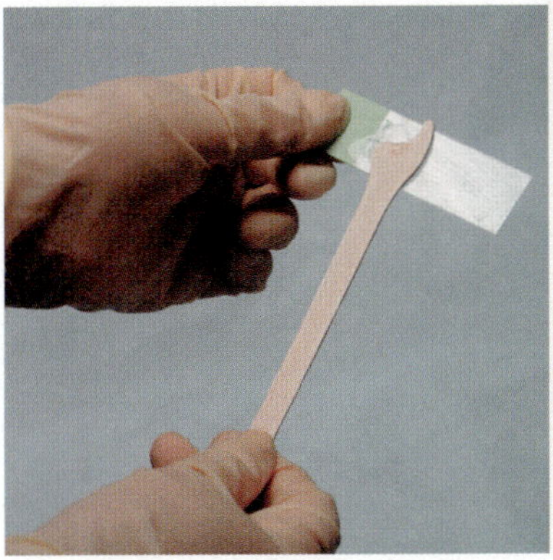

b.

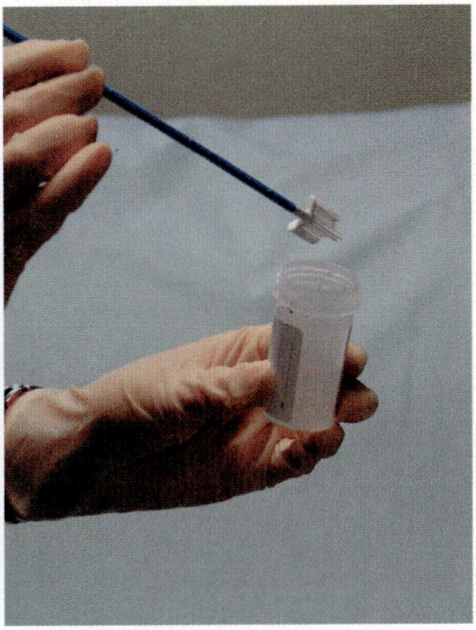

图 8 a. 将涂片抹在显微玻片上。b. 液基细胞学样本
a. Spreading the smear on a microscope slide. b. Specimen for liquid based cytology

阴道镜

适应证

宫颈涂片检查显示无自发好转的交界性改变或轻度核异常，或单次涂片检查显示中、重度核异常的妇女，都应进行阴道镜检查。

描述

阴道镜（图10）是一个双筒的显微镜。可以获得清晰的宫颈三维图像，放大倍数在6～40倍（图11）。这一技术既可确定引起宫颈涂片异常的严重程度又可确定其在宫颈上的位置，使临床医师可以评估局部烧蚀治疗的可行性。

方法

患者取截石位，使用双瓣窥器暴露宫颈。干棉球清除宫颈黏液，用 5% 醋酸将异常区域染白（醋酸白）。如果移行带的上界位于宫颈管内，使用钳子可帮助暴露整个区域（图 12）。如果移行带的上界不能见到，那么这样的检查是不完全的。这种情况在25岁或更年轻的妇女中发生率低于10%，但是在40岁以上的妇女发生率大于 30%。

应用活检钳从阴道镜下异常区域取样以确定组织学诊断。结果回报后，可用Semm电凝或激光的烧蚀治疗。对移行带进行的电圈切除（diathermy loop excision，DLE）可用来切除宫颈病灶。对于中度或重度核异常涂片以及阴道镜改变与之相一致的妇女，治疗过程中切除了异常，得到了好样本用于组织学分析，这样在一次访视中使该病能被评估和治疗（访问和治疗）。

Colposcopy

Indications

All women who have had cervical smears showing borderline changes or mild dyskaryosis that does not resolve spontaneously, or those women with a single smear showing moderately or severely dyskaryotic cells, should be referred for colposcopy.

Description

The colposcope (Fig. 10) is a binocular microscope. An illuminated, three-dimensional view of the cervix is obtained, magnified between 6 and 40 times (Fig. 11). This technique identifies both the severity of the abnormality giving rise to an abnormal smear and also its position on the cervix. Hence it allows the clinician to assess the suitability for local ablative therapy.

Technique

The patient is examined in the lithotomy position and a bivalve speculum is used to expose the cervix. Cotton wool swabs are then used to clean mucus off the cervix before applying 5% acetic acid to stain the abnormal areas white (acetowhite). If the upper limit of the transformation zone lies within the endocervical canal, forceps may be useful in exposing the whole area (Fig. 12). If the upper limit of the transformation zone cannot be visualized then the examination must be considered incomplete. This occurs in less than 10% of women aged 25 years or less, but in more than 30% of women over the age of 40 years.

Punch biopsy forceps can be used to obtain a sample from colposcopically abnormal areas to make a histological diagnosis. Once the results of this are known, ablative treatment such as Semm cautery or laser can be applied. Diathermy loop excision (DLE) of the transformation zone is used to excise cervical lesions. For women with moderate or severely dyskaryotic smears and colposcopic changes consistent with this, the treatment process removes the abnormality and produces a good sample for histological analysis, thus enabling assessment and treatment at one visit (see and treat).

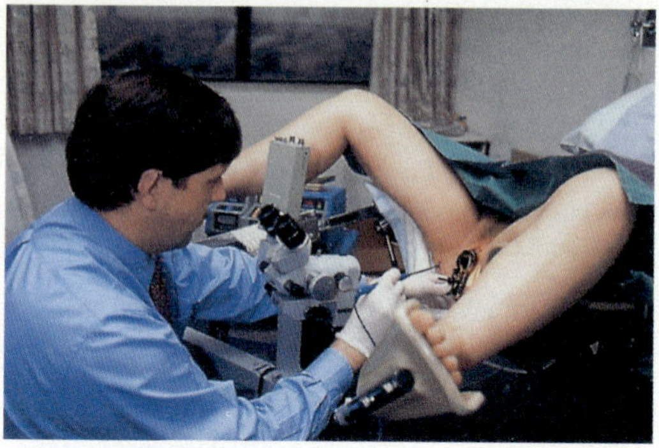

图 10 临床阴道镜
Colposcopy clinic

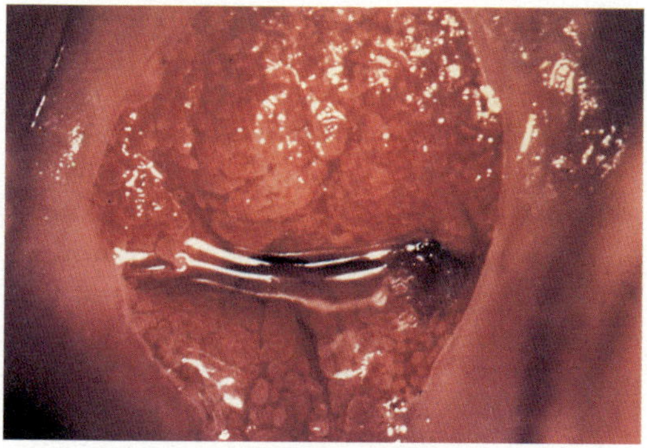

图 11 正常宫颈的阴道镜图像
Colpophotograph of a normal cervix

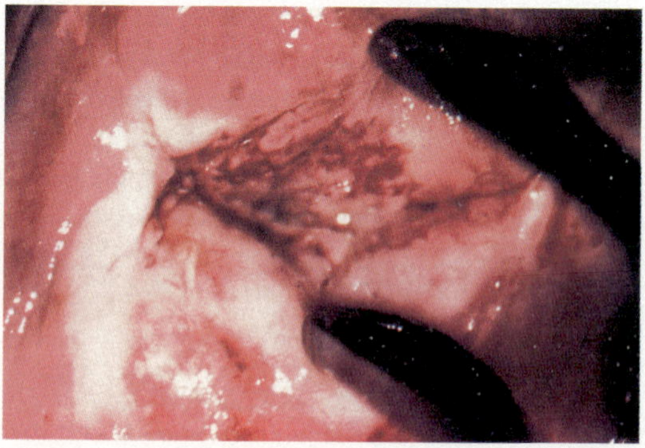

图 12 暴露鳞柱交界
Exposing the squamocolumnar junction

超声

描述

当声波从解剖结构中反射回来时，超声波图像检查可以记录高频率声波。超声波是机械波，它超出听觉的范围。当把超声向不同密度的介质发射时，声波就会以不同速度传播。回声产生于这些介质之间的表面，密度差异越大，产生的回声强度越大。回声信号被测量，并且转化成检查区域的临床图像。因此，要想有一个好的成像，必须有一个无气隙的紧密接触腹部的换能探头。超声是一种简单、无痛苦、无副作用的操作。超声医师和患者能够一同看到超声图像（图 13）。

多种探头可供使用（图 14）。如用腹部探头，膀胱充盈形成超声“窗”。如用阴道探头，无须膀胱充盈，在早孕中非常有用。

适应证

超声几乎可用于检查任何的盆腔异常，因为所有的结构可通常经阴道或腹部扫描显示出来。通过应用彩色多普勒技术能够显示血液流到不同器官（图 15）。

宫内妊娠最初的迹象能够在妊娠第 5 周被探测到，显示为一个小的轮廓锐利的腔，被称为妊娠囊。妊娠第7～8周，胚胎结构表现为独特的回声。如果应用经阴道探头，妊娠第5周即可看到胎儿心脏跳动。

Ultrasound

Description

Ultrasonography records high-frequency sound waves as they are reflected from anatomic structures. Ultrasound waves are mechanical waves beyond the scope of hearing. When they are directed toward media of differing densities, the sound waves spread out with differing velocities. Echoes arise at the interfaces between these media, and the greater the density differences the greater the intensity of the echoes. This echo signal is measured and converted into a clinical picture of the area under examination. Thus, for good visualization there must be an air-free coupling of the transducer to the abdomen. Ultrasound is a simple and painless procedure that has no known ill-effects. The ultrasonographer and patient can look at the ultrasound image together (Fig. 13).

Various probes are now available (Fig. 14). If an abdominal probe is used, the scan is performed with a full bladder which provides a sonographic 'window'. A vaginal probe eliminates the need to have a full bladder, which is especially useful in early pregnancy.

Indications

Ultrasonography is useful in almost any pelvic abnormality as all structures can usually be demonstrated either by transvaginal or abdominal scanning. Blood flow to various organs can be demonstrated using Colour Doppler techniques (Fig. 15).

The first sign of an intrauterine pregnancy can be detected in the 5th week as a small, sharply outlined cavity which is the gestational sac. Between the 7th and 8th weeks, embryonic structures can be visualized as distinct echoes. The fetal heart can be seen beating from 5 weeks if a transvaginal probe is used.

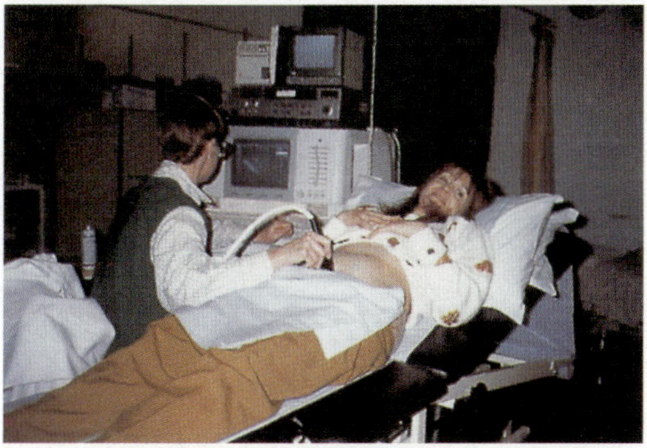

图 13　正在进行腹部超声检查
An abdominal ultrasound being performed

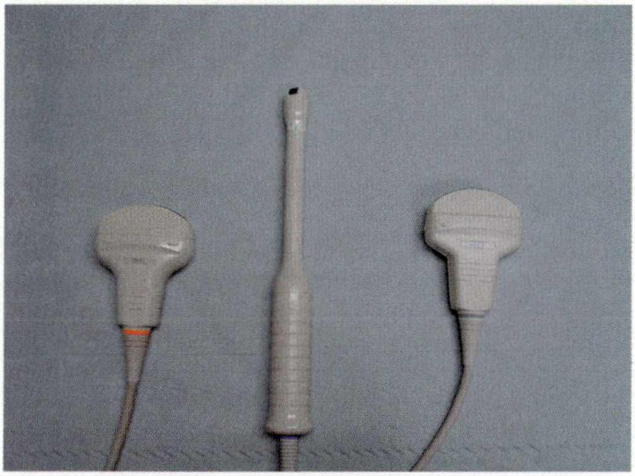

图 14　阴道和腹部的超声探头
Vaginal and abdominal ultrasound probes

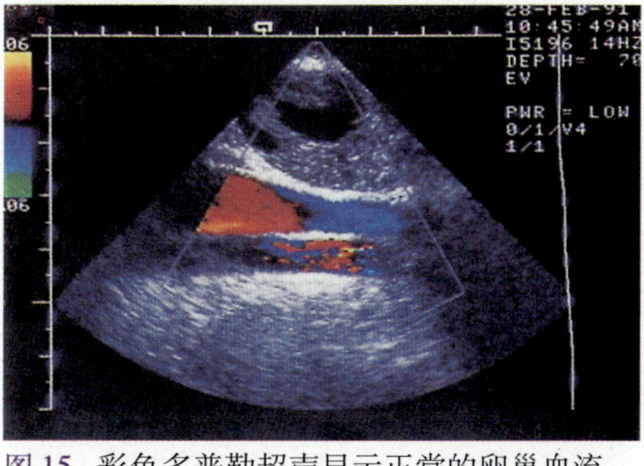

图 15　彩色多普勒超声显示正常的卵巢血流
Colour Doppler ultrasound illustrating normal ovarian blood flow

子宫输卵管造影

描述

子宫输卵管造影（hysterosalpingography，HSG）是一种用来评估输卵管是否通畅及显示宫腔结构异常的 X 线诊断方法。

适应证

HSG会显示输卵管是否通畅，如不通畅则可以找到阻塞的部位。但这种方法不能显示盆腔的情况，例如输卵管周围粘连和/或骨盆畸形，它们可导致生育能力受损，即使输卵管是通畅的。

技术

HSG无须麻醉，在X线科室完成。应用双瓣窥器暴露宫颈，将套管插入宫颈使不透射线的染色剂注入宫腔。应用影像增强器观察此过程，并在胶片上显像（图 16）。

HyCoSy（子宫输卵管对比超声检查）

另一种可供选择的探测输卵管通畅程度的技术，是将产生回声的悬浮液注入宫腔，在超声监护下悬浮液流入输卵管（图 17）。

Hysterosalpingography

Description

Hysterosalpingography (HSG) is an X-ray method of assessing fallopian tube patency and demonstrating structural abnormalities of the uterine cavity.

Indications

HSG will show whether the fallopian tubes are patent. If not, the area in which the tubes are blocked can be identified. It will not give information concerning the condition of the pelvis, i.e. the presence of peritubular adhesions and/or pelvic distortion which may impair fertility even though the tubes are patent.

Technique

HSG is usually performed without anaesthetic in the X-ray department. A bivalve speculum is used to expose the cervix which is cannulated to enable radiopaque dye to be injected into the uterine cavity. The procedure is viewed using an image intensifier and recorded on film (Fig. 16).

HyCoSy (hysterosalpingo contrast sonography)

An alternative technique to assess tubal patency whereby an echogenic suspension is inserted into the uterine cavity, which then flows through the tubes under ultrasonic surveillance (Fig. 17).

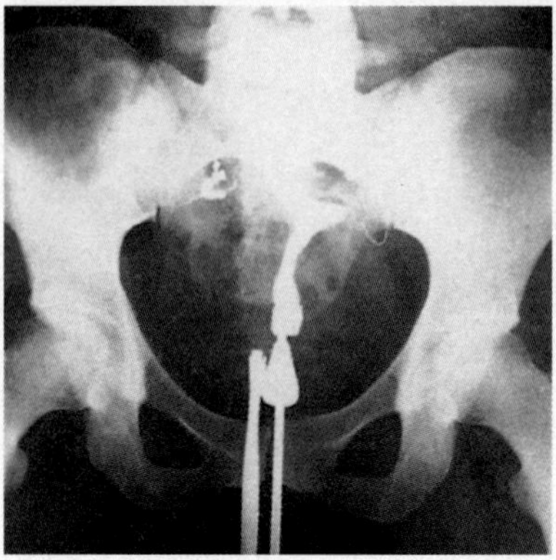

图 16　子宫输卵管造影显像子宫和输卵管结构
Hysterosalpingogram outlining the uterine and tubal anatomy

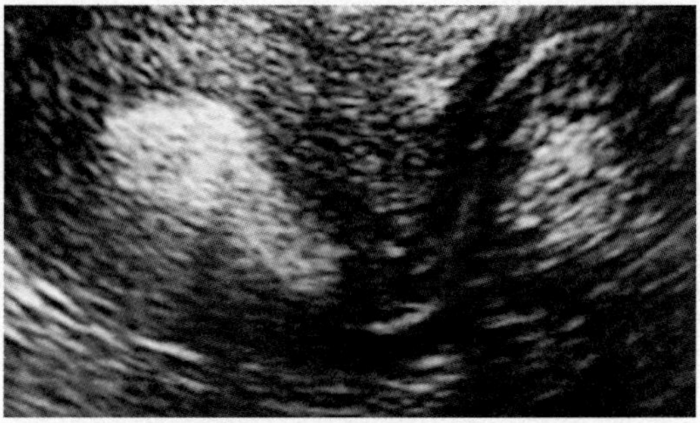

图 17　子宫输卵管对比超声（HyCoSy）
Hysterosalpingo contrast sonography (HyCoSy)

宫腔镜

描述与技术 宫腔镜检查是一种可视的宫腔检查。宫腔镜是一种由护套包绕的内镜。患者在全麻或局麻下取截石位，将宫腔镜通过宫颈插入宫腔内。

适应证 在宫腔镜下可以看到子宫内膜息肉、纤维瘤、粘连以及不同类型的子宫内膜，例如正常的、增生的、萎缩的、恶变的子宫内膜（图18 ~ 20）。还可使用宫腔镜进行内膜活检、分离粘连、取出息肉及异位的节育器。月经过多的妇女可用电切环或激光切除子宫内膜内层，黏膜下肌瘤也可用此方法切除。

并发症 这一操作的并发症包括子宫穿孔、感染和液体负荷过多（例如内膜切除时应用膨宫介质）。

Hysteroscopy

Description and technique

Hysteroscopy is a method that enables visual examination of the uterine cavity. A hysteroscope is a telescope surrounded by a sheath. It is inserted into the uterine cavity through the cervix with the patient in the lithotomy position and under either local or general anaesthesia.

Indications

Endometrial polyps, fibroids and adhesions within the uterine cavity can be visualized hysteroscopically, together with different types of endometrium, e.g. normal, hyperplastic, atrophic and malignant (Figs 18~20). It is also possible to use the hysteroscope to take endometrial biopsies, divide adhesions, and remove polyps and misplaced IUCDs. The endometrial lining can be removed using an electrical resection loop or laser in women with menorrhagia. Submucous fibroids can also be removed in this way.

Complications

Complications of the procedure include perforation of the uterus, infection and fluid overload (e.g. if fluid distension medium is used for endometrial resection).

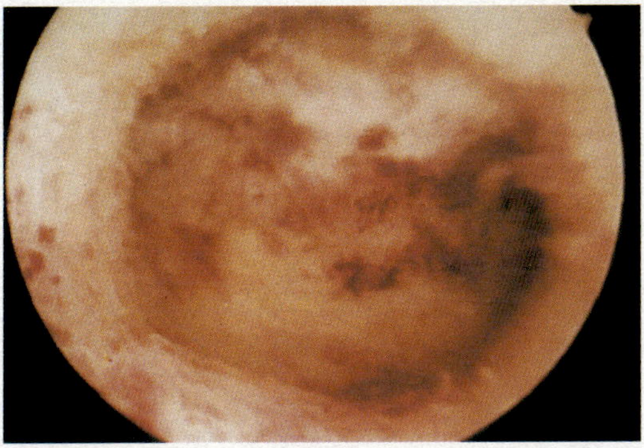

图 18　正常的子宫内膜
Normal endometrium

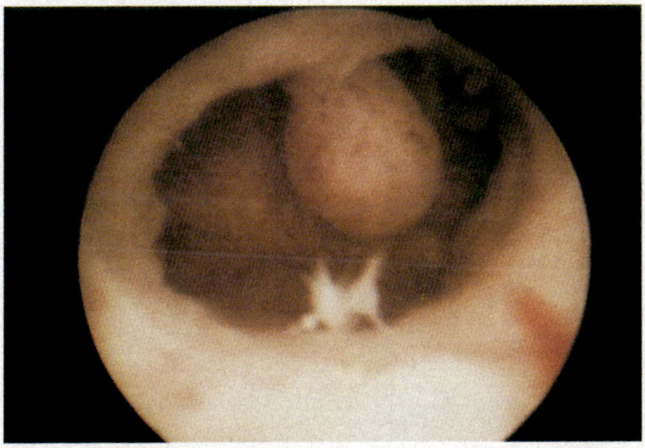

图 19　内膜息肉
Endometrial polyp

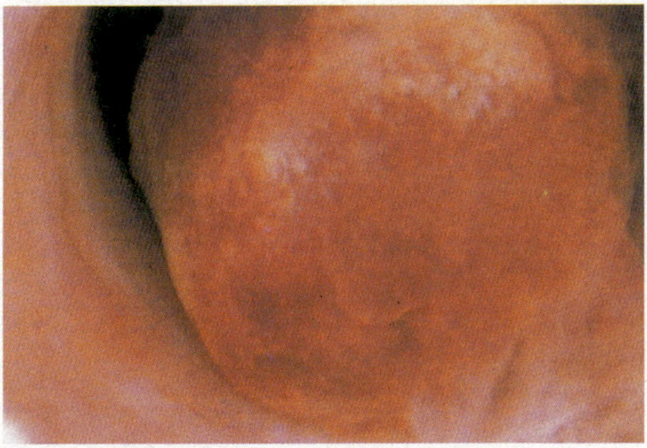

图 20　带蒂肌瘤
Endometrial pedunculated fibroid

腹腔镜

描述

在本质上腹腔镜是一种内镜，在腹腔充满CO_2气体后插入腹腔。腹腔镜使得妇科疾病的诊断和手术在非剖腹手术情况下完成成为可能（图 21，22）。

技术

常常在全麻下进行，患者被麻醉及给予人工通气。病人采用改良的Lloyd-Davies体位，头部向下。膀胱留置尿管。在脐部做一小开口，将气腹针插入腹腔，CO_2气体充填腹腔至压力达20mmHg。把针退出，置入腹腔镜的套针及插管，取出套针，插入腹腔镜，直视盆腔器官（图 23）。如需要，可在腹腔镜直视下于耻骨弓上或者一侧髂窝插管，以允许盆腔脏器的操作以及为各种手术置入器械。

适应证

包括盆腔痛、异位妊娠的诊断和治疗、不孕症的检查、绝育术、创伤、节育器异位、辅助受孕以及妇科癌症的分期，包括盆腔淋巴结取样。更进一步的操作包括腹腔镜辅助的阴式子宫切除术（laparoscopically assisted vaginal hysterectomy, LAVH）、腹腔镜下阴道悬吊以及腹腔镜下骶骨阴道固定术。

并发症

这一操作的并发症包括:

- 疼痛，尤其是由 CO_2 刺激膈肌引起的肩部顶端疼痛
- 出血
- 膀胱、肠管穿孔
- 气体注入异位
- 死亡率大概在 1∶15 000

Laparoscopy

Description

The laparoscope is essentially a telescope that is inserted into the abdominal cavity after it has been inflated with carbon-dioxide. The direct view obtained allows the diagnosis of gynaecological disorders and surgery (Figs 21, 22) without laparotomy.

Technique

The procedure is almost invariably performed under general anaesthesia with the patient paralysed and ventilated. The patient is placed in the modified Lloyd-Davies position with the head down. The bladder is catheterized. A small incision is made at the umbilicus and a Veress needle is inserted into the peritoneal cavity. Carbon dioxide is insufflated into the peritoneal cavity to a pressure of 20 mmHg. The needle is withdrawn and the laparoscopic trocar and cannula are inserted. The trocar is withdrawn and replaced with the laparoscope, which allows direct visualization of the pelvic organs (Fig. 23). If needed, further cannulae are inserted under direct laparoscopic vision, suprapubically or in either iliac fossa, to permit manipulation of pelvic organs and instrumentation for various surgical techniques.

Indications

These include pelvic pain, diagnosis and treatment of ectopic pregnancy, infertility investigation, sterilization, trauma, lost IUCD and assisted conception techniques, as well as staging procedures for gynaecological cancer, including pelvic lymph node sampling. More advanced procedures include laparoscopically assisted vaginal hysterectomy (LAVH), laparoscopic colposuspension and laparoscopic sacrocolpopexy.

Complications

Complications of the procedure include:

- Pain, especially shoulder-tip pain from CO_2 diaphragmatic irritation
- Bleeding
- Puncture of bladder, bowel
- Misplacement of gas
- Mortality rate approximately 1 in 15 000.

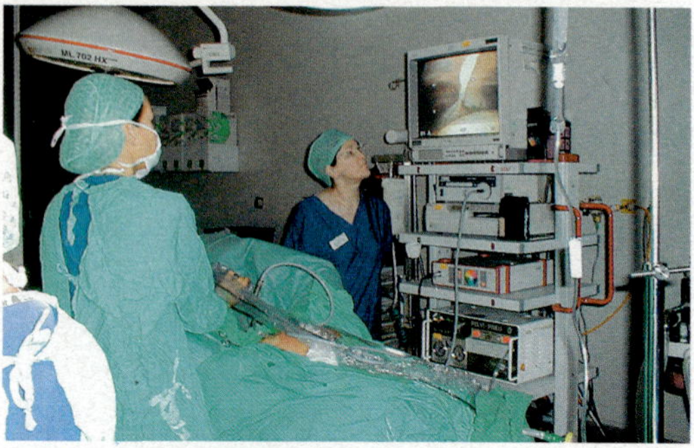

图 21　进行腹腔镜操作
Laparoscopy being performed

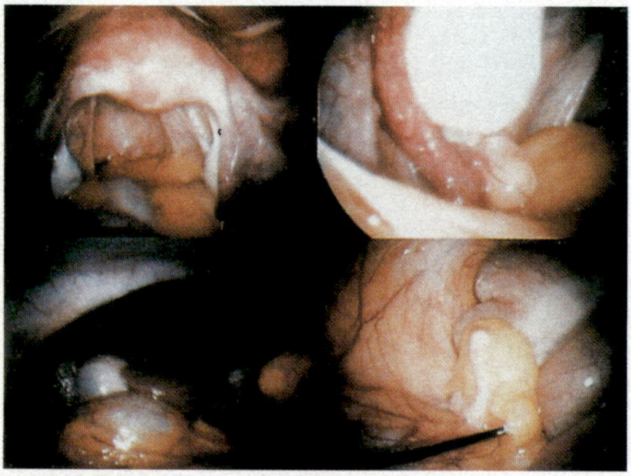

图 22　腹腔镜下观察内脏
Laparoscopic views of internal organs

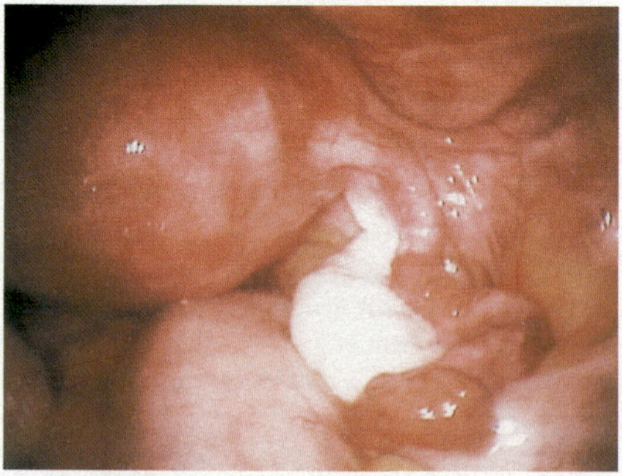

图 23　腹腔镜下正常的输卵管和卵巢
Normal fallopian tube and ovary as seen with laparoscopy

先天性疾病

阴道积液

发生该疾病时，闭锁膜刚好位于处女膜上。在梗阻部位以上积液使阴道膨胀（图 24）。新生儿阴道积液可表现为尿潴留、腹痛，如大量积液时可有下腹包块。治疗方法是单纯把闭锁膜切开放液。

阴道积血

阴道积血的情形与阴道积液相同，只是阴道积血发生在青春期后。月经血不能排出而集聚在闭锁的处女膜之上，使阴道膨胀明显甚至子宫也发生膨胀。症状可表现为腹部疼痛、尿潴留或大的腹部包块。外阴检查可见需要切开的淡蓝色膨胀突出的膜。

阴唇融合

阴唇彼此相互粘连（图 25），使得看上去好像阴道缺如。病因不清，可能与雌激素水平过低有关。应用雌激素软膏 10 ~ 14 天后通常会自行分开。

Congenital

Hydrocolpos

In this disorder, an imperforate membrane is situated immediately above the hymen. Above this obstruction the vagina can become distended by fluid (Fig. 24). Hydrocolpos can present in the neonate as retention of urine, abdominal pain and a lower abdominal swelling if there is a large quantity of fluid. The treatment is simple incision of the membrane to release the fluid.

Haematocolpos

The same situation as in hydrocolpos occurs in haematocolpos, except that the problem does not arise until puberty. The menstrual fluid is unable to be released and collects above the imperforate hymen, grossly expanding the vagina and even the uterus. The presenting symptoms may include abdominal pain, urinary retention or a large abdominal mass. Vulval inspection will reveal a bulging bluish membrane that requires incision.

Fused labia

The labia minora become adherent to each other (Fig. 25), and it may appear as though the vagina is absent. The aetiology is not known, but the condition is probably due to low oestrogen levels. Application of oestrogen cream usually results in spontaneous separation after 10~14 days.

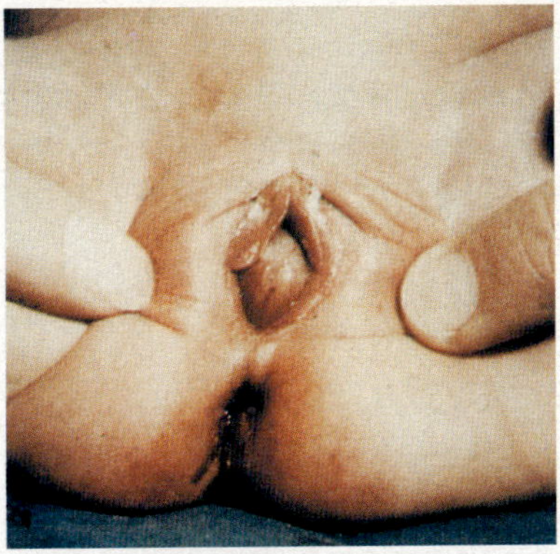

图 24 阴道积液
Hydrocolpos

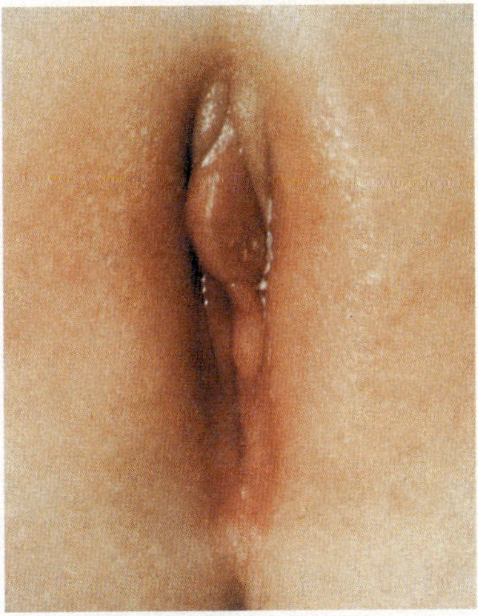

图 25 阴唇融合
Fused labia

先天畸形

苗勒管发育成输卵管、子宫、阴道的上2/3，阴道下1/3 来自尿生殖窦。胚胎发育过程中可产生各种缺陷（图 26）。包括下列发育的失败:

- 发育过程中的异常，例如无中肾旁管
- 副中肾管穿通
- 副中肾管融合
- 中隔退失（图 27）
- 穹窿底部发育
- 副中肾管与尿生殖窦融合
- 中肾旁系统与尿生殖窦之间横隔退失

幼童时期疾病

外阴阴道炎

这是儿童最常见的妇科疾病。使未成熟阴道易于感染的原因有三种:

- 缺乏保护性的酸性分泌物
- 粪便和碎屑的污染
- 免疫机能受损

细菌学检查结果一般为混合感染，儿童会主诉外阴疼痛、异常分泌物或排尿痛，线虫感染有时也会引起这种情况。

异物

这些异物经常会引起脓性分泌物或流血。

葡萄状肉瘤

儿童时期肿瘤少见，但以胚胎性横纹肌肉瘤最为严重。外表常呈葡萄簇状（图 28），但也可表现为息肉。肿瘤在阴道或宫颈阴道部的上皮下组织中广泛播散。在行扩大的子宫切除术或阴道切除术前通常应化疗（图 29）。

Congenital abnormalities

The müllerian ducts are the embryological precursors of the fallopian tubes, uterus and upper two-thirds of the vagina. The lower one-third of the vagina develops from the urogenital sinus. Various defects can occur during embryological development (Fig. 26). These include failure of:

- development, e.g. no paramesonephric duct
- paramesonephric duct canalization
- fusion of paramesonephric ducts
- median septum loss (Fig. 27)
- fundal dome development
- fusion of paramesonephric ducts with urogenital sinus
- transverse septum loss between paramesonephric system and urogenital sinus.

Problems in early childhood

Vulvovaginitis

This is the most common gynaecological problem in children. There are three factors that make the immature vagina susceptible to infection:

- lack of protective acid secretion
- contamination by stool and debris
- impaired mechanisms of immunity.

The usual bacteriological finding is of mixed bacterial flora. The child will complain of vulval soreness, discharge, or pain on micturition. Threadworm infestation can sometimes cause this condition.

Foreign bodies

These usually produce a purulent discharge or bleeding.

Botryoid sarcoma

Tumours are rare in childhood but embryonal rhabdomyosarcoma is the most serious. It is often grapelike in appearance (Fig. 28) but may appear simply as a polyp. The tumour spreads extensively in the subepithelial tissues of the vagina or ectocervix. Chemotherapy is generally given prior to extended hysterectomy or vaginectomy (Fig. 29).

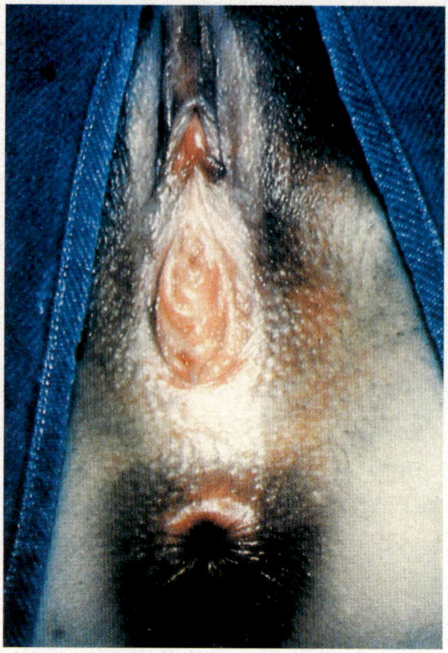

图 26　无阴道——一种先天性缺陷
Absent vagina — a congenital defect

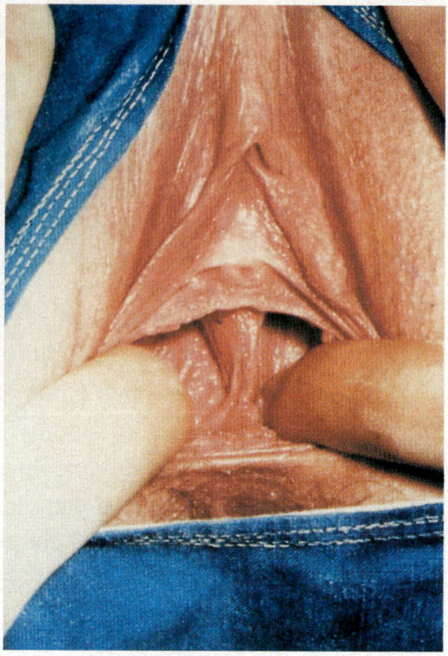

图 27　阴道纵隔
Vaginal septum

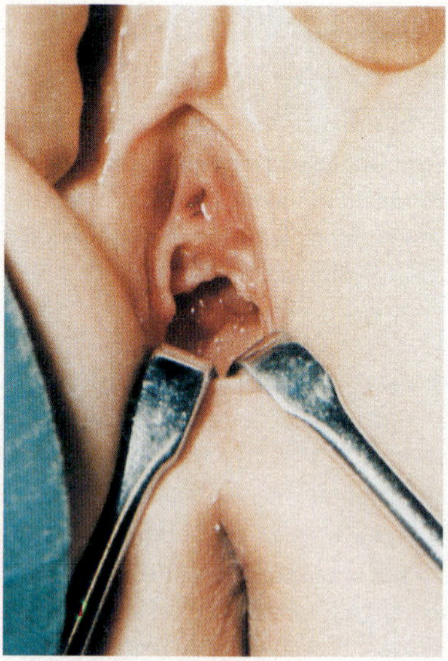

图 28　葡萄状肉瘤
Botryoid sarcoma at examination

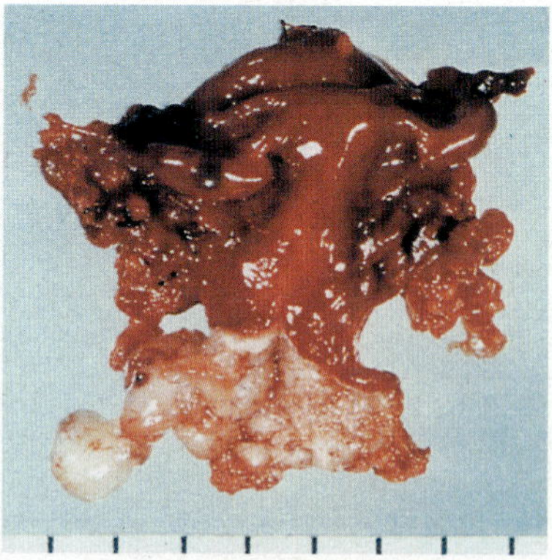

图 29　葡萄状肉瘤的手术标本
Surgical specimen of botryoid sarcoma

性虐待

受到性虐待的儿童受到身体和心理上的创伤。当怀疑有性虐待时，必须由有经验的妇科医生进行彻底的检查。必须采集宫颈、阴道、肛门的拭子标本检查性传播疾病，同样应采集精液标本。如果有可能的话应照相，并且准确记录所受的创伤。检查通常是在麻醉下完成的。

外阴裂伤很常见，处女膜通常破裂（图 30），必须检查是否有肛门裂伤（图31）及扩张，在身体的其他部位也要寻找擦伤或其他的外伤表现。还应考虑是否有骨折。这些儿童通常需要入院治疗，直至将家庭状况彻底调查清楚。通常采用由社会工作者、儿科医生、妇科医生组成的多学科方法。

女性生殖器阉割

这种风俗仍在进行，主要在非洲。在英国则是非法的。这一操作的程度有不同差异，可单纯切除小阴唇边缘，直至完全切除阴唇及阴蒂并缝合阴道口。并发症很常见，如果手术在接近青春期时进行，可有严重的出血和脓毒症。当完成整个阴唇的切除后，用带子将大腿绑住使切口对合，并在两边缘之间插一只小棍引流尿液。导致的严重瘢痕使尿道口及前庭被遮蔽（图32）。还可导致皮样囊肿（图33），使尿流改变方向，引起周围皮肤及阴道慢性感染。几乎不能完成性交，可能必须分开皮肤桥。若阴道分娩，前方会阴切开可能是必须的。梗阻性难产时，停留在阴道内过久的胎儿引起阴道壁压迫性坏死。

Sexual abuse

Children who have been sexually abused endure physical and psychological trauma. When sexual abuse is suspected, a thorough examination must be carried out by an experienced gynaecologist. Swabs for sexually transmitted diseases must be taken from the vagina, cervix and anus. Samples for semen should also be taken. Photographs should be taken if possible, and the signs of physical trauma should be accurately documented. The examinations are often performed under anaesthesia.

Vulval bruising is common, and the hymen is often perforated (Fig. 30). Anal bruising must be looked for (Fig. 31), and anal dilatation. The rest of the body must be searched for bruising or other signs of trauma. Fractures should be suspected. These children usually need to be admitted until the domestic situation has been thoroughly investigated. A multidisciplinary approach involving social workers, paediatricians and gynaecologists is usually adopted.

Female genital mutilation

This custom is still practised, mainly in Africa. It is illegal in the UK. The extent of the procedure varies from trimming of the labia minora to complete removal of the labia and clitoris with sewing over of the vaginal introitus. Complications are common. If the operation is carried out near puberty, haemorrhage and sepsis can be severe. When complete excision of the labia and minora is performed, the denuded edges are encouraged to unite by strapping the thighs together, with a stick between the edges to allow passage of urine. The resulting scarring can be extreme and the urethra and vestibule hidden (Fig. 32). Epidermoid cysts can result (Fig. 33). This deflects the urinary stream causing chronic infection both of the surrounding skin and vagina. Intercourse may be impossible, and division of a skin bridge may be necessary. For vaginal delivery, an anterior episiotomy may be necessary. In obstructed labour, the fetus may be in the vagina for long enough to cause vaginal wall pressure necrosis.

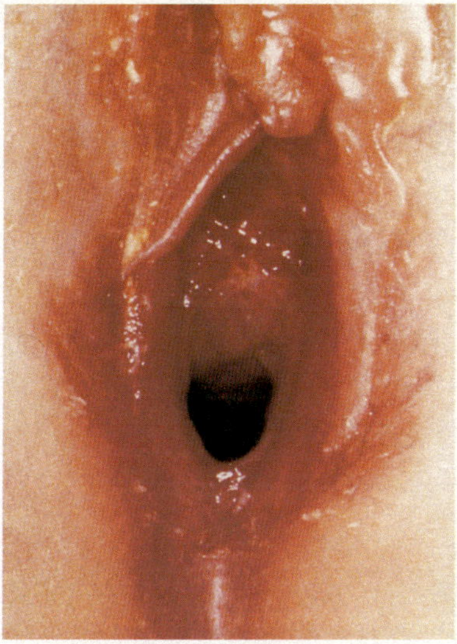

图 30 阴道和外阴擦伤
Vaginal and vulval bruising

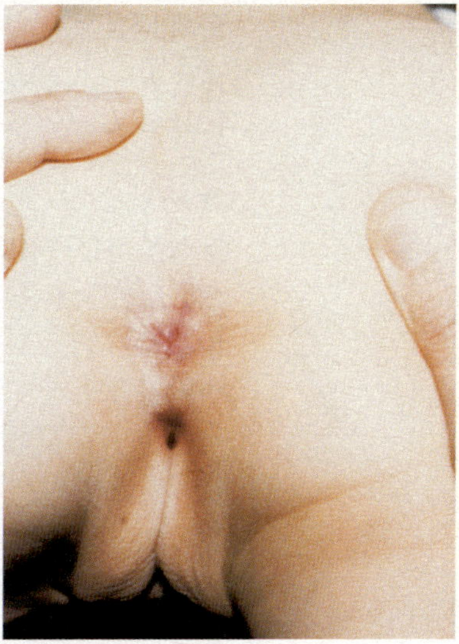

图 31 肛门创伤
Anal trauma

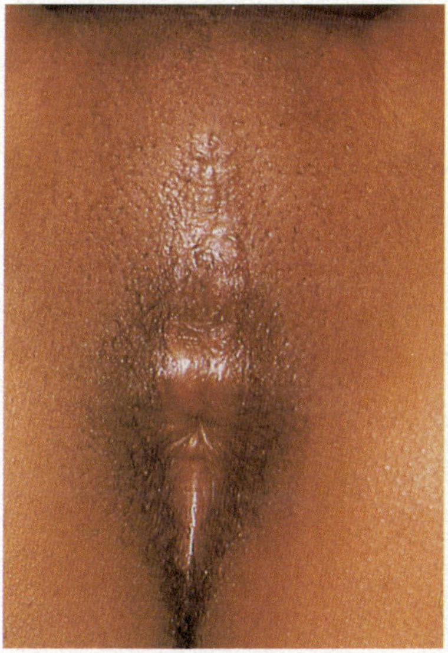

图 32 女性生殖器阉割
Female genital mutilation

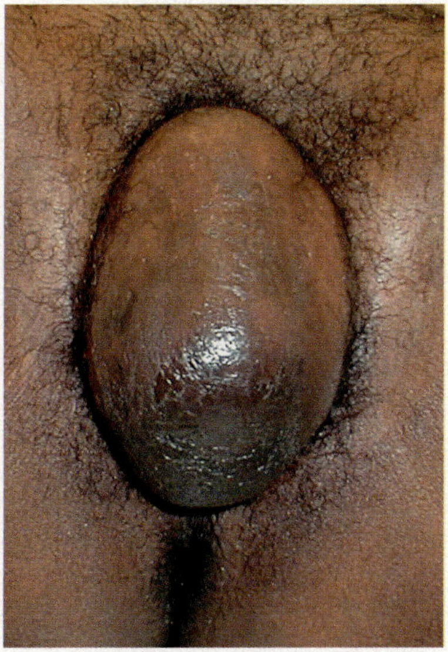

图 33 女性生殖器阉割引起的皮样囊肿
An epidermoid cyst as a result of female genital mutilation

青春期疾病

在青春期激素变化很复杂。功能异常能够揭示在儿童时期表现不明显的染色体、酶及结构的异常。

特纳综合征

特纳综合征（图34）患者缺少一条性染色体，这样会导致卵巢性不孕，表现为原发性闭经、身材矮小和性器官幼稚型。雄激素受体缺陷而有正常XY者则会男性化发育失败而有正常女性外观，乳腺发育良好。原发性闭经可能是睾丸女性化最早的表现（图 35）。

5α 还原酶缺乏

5α 还原酶缺乏（图 36）导致男性基因型的孩子外生殖器男性化失败。而在青春期产生大量睾酮，正常的睾丸内陷，呈假女性雄性化。应行睾丸切除，并且给予雌激素替代治疗以确保其女性表型。

其他问题有青春期早熟，表现为乳房发育及月经来潮提前；或因下丘脑病理性成熟延迟引起的青春期滞后。

两性畸形

定义

两性畸形是个体的染色体、性腺、内生殖器与性别表型或抚养的性别不一致。

临床特征

出生时由于存在模棱两可的外生殖器而被发现（图37），儿童时期由于青春期早熟或青春期由于青春期改变与假定性别不相符，或者由于没有出现青春期而被诊断。

Disorders of puberty

The hormonal changes of puberty are complex. Disordered function can reveal chromosomal, enzymatic and structural abnormalities not obvious in childhood.

Turner's syndrome

In Turner's syndrome (Fig. 34), the absence of the one sex chromosome leads to ovarian dysgenesis resulting in primary amenorrhoea, short stature and sexual infantilism. Alternatively, androgen-receptor defects with a normal XY complement lead to failure of masculinization and apparently normal, full breast development. Primary amenorrhoea may be the first presentation of testicular feminization (Fig. 35).

5α reductase deficiency

In 5α reductase deficiency (Fig. 36), the lack of the enzyme likewise results in failure of masculinization of the external genitalia in the genotypic male child. However, at puberty the large increase in testosterone production by normal, internalized testes results in androgenization of the presumed female. The testes are removed and oestrogen replacement ensures a phenotypic female.

Other problems include precocious puberty, as indicated by early thelarche or menarche, or delayed puberty where hypothalamic maturation is pathologically late.

Intersex

Definition

An intersex is an individual in whom there is discordance between chromosomal, gonadal, internal genital and phenotype sex, or the sex of rearing.

Clinical features

It may be declared at birth because of ambiguous external genitalia (Fig. 37), during childhood because of precocious puberty or during adolescence because pubertal changes are inappropriate to presumed gender, or because puberty fails to occur.

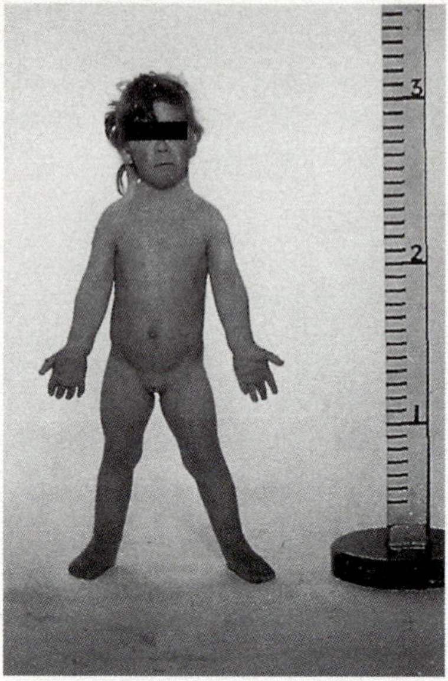

图 34 特纳综合征
Turner's syndrome

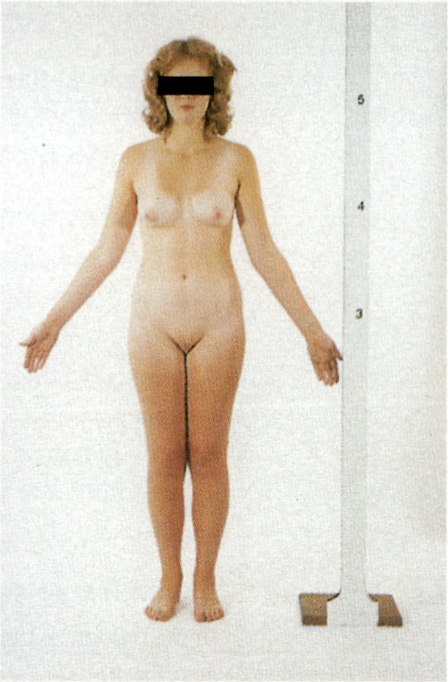

图 35 睾丸女性化
Testicular feminization

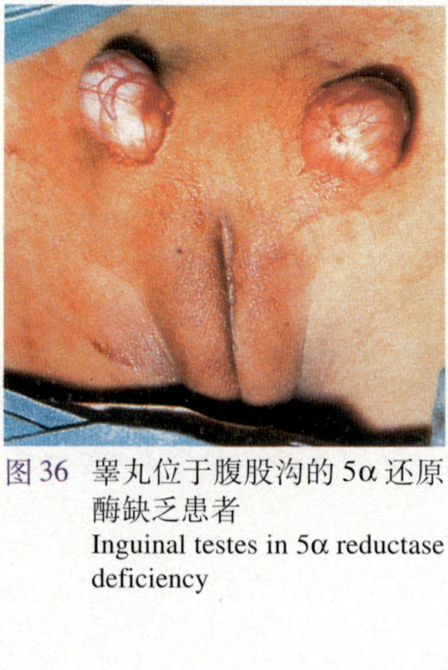

图 36 睾丸位于腹股沟的 5α 还原酶缺乏患者
Inguinal testes in 5α reductase deficiency

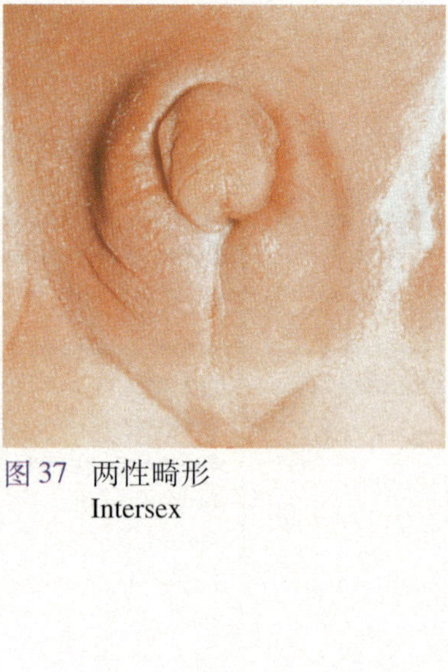

图 37 两性畸形
Intersex

青春期

在青春期下丘脑-垂体-卵巢轴发生改变，下丘脑分泌 GnRH 呈脉冲式。GnRH 刺激垂体前叶脉冲式释放FSH与LH。因此，在周期中FSH与LH每70—220分钟（取决于周期时相）脉冲式分泌一次。卵巢激素通过对下丘脑及垂体的反馈作用影响促性腺激素的释放。

激素变化

在每个周期开始时（图 38a），FSH 刺激卵泡发育，其中一个卵泡成为优势卵泡，而其他卵泡闭锁。优势卵泡分泌的雌激素增加，会引起血中雌二醇水平升高，触发垂体分泌LH高峰，从而引起排卵。LH峰又刺激卵泡分泌孕酮及前列腺素。卵泡释放卵母细胞后萎缩，成为释放孕酮的黄体。如果没有妊娠，黄体将于 10 日后萎缩。如妊娠，HCG 将维持黄体激素分泌直至妊娠十周。

子宫内膜变化

子宫内膜在月经周期的前半部分（图 38b）受雌激素的刺激发生腺体增生及内膜增厚。在月经周期后半部分，孕激素的分泌引起腺体内层上皮转化为空泡，腺体及螺旋动脉继续增长。间质出现水肿并蜕膜化。

雌孕激素水平的下降引起循环障碍和螺旋动脉扩张，最终导致广泛的血管阻塞、局部缺血与细胞崩解，导致溶酶体酶的释放。来自下一个卵泡的雌激素升高会阻止进一步的破坏。宫颈与阴道显示与卵巢皮质类固醇激素分泌相应的变化（图 39）。

4 The menstrual cycle

Puberty

At puberty the HPO axis changes and GnRH is secreted in a pulsatile fashion from the hypothalamus. This stimulates a pulsatile release of FSH and LH from the anterior pituitary. Thereafter, FSH and LH are secreted in pulses every 70-220 min depending on the cycle phase. The release of the gonadotrophins is regulated by the ovarian steroid feedback on the hypothalamus and pituitary.

Hormonal changes

At the beginning of each cycle (Fig. 38a), FSH stimulates growth in follicles, with one follicle becoming dominant while the others undergo atresia. Oestrogen production in the dominant follicle increases, leading to rising estradiol blood levels, which trigger the LH surge from the pituitary, in turn causing ovulation. This LH surge also stimulates the production of progesterone and prostaglandins in the follicle. The oocyte is then released from the follicle, which shrinks and becomes the progesterone-producing corpus luteum. Unless a pregnancy occurs, this regresses after about 10 days. If pregnancy occurs, the HCG maintains the production of steroids from the corpus luteum until week 10 of pregnancy.

Endometrial changes

The endometrium in the first half of the cycle (Fig. 38b) responds to the oestrogenic stimulation by growth of the glands and endometrial thickening. When progesterone is produced in the second half of the cycle, the epithelium lining the glands develops vacuoles, and the glands and the spiral arterioles continue to grow. The stroma becomes oedematous and undergoes decidualization.

Falling levels of oestrogen and progesterone cause cyclical constriction and dilatation of the spiral arterioles; eventually generalized vasoconstriction, ischaemia and cell disintegration occur leading to release of lysosomal enzymes. Breakdown is halted by rising levels of oestrogen from the next follicle. The cervix and vagina show changes in response to ovarian steroid output (Fig. 39).

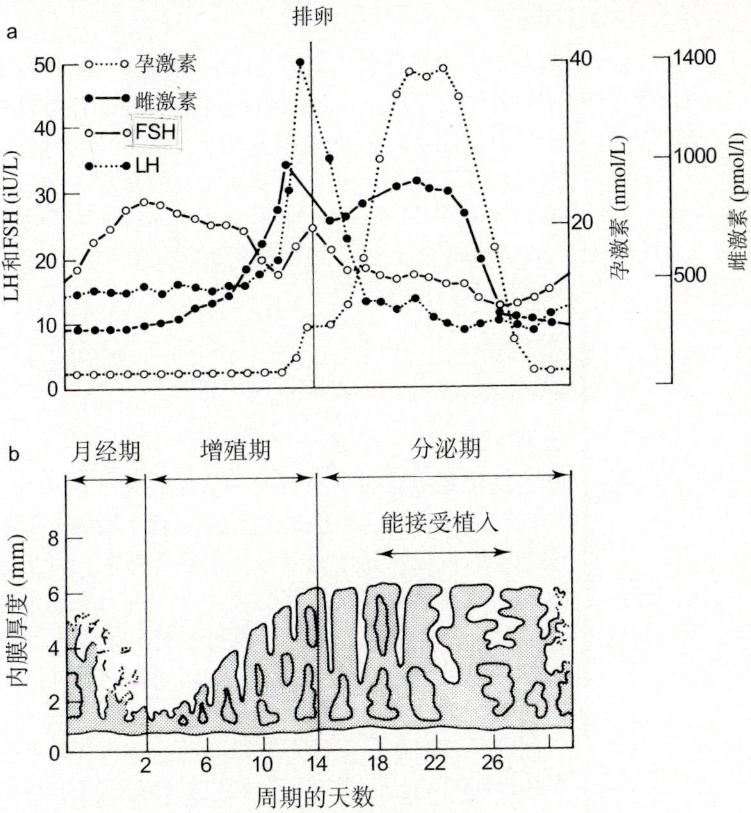

图 38　月经周期。a. 激素改变。b. 内膜改变
The menstrual cycle. a. Hormonal changes. b. Endometrial changes

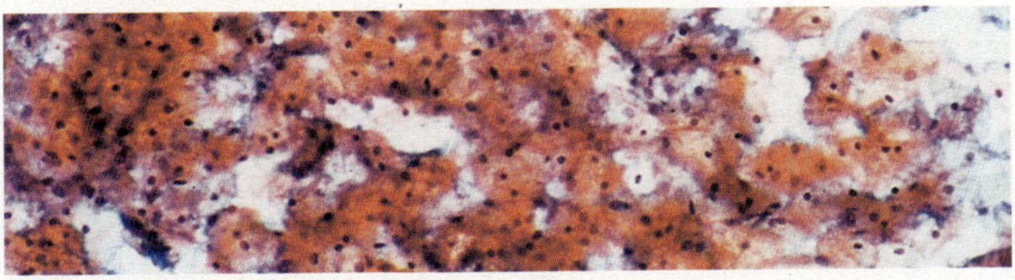

图 39　阴道细胞学检查显示雌激素刺激
Vaginal cytology showing oestrogenic stimulation

闭经

闭经定义为无月经，可分为原发性闭经（无月经来潮）及继发性闭经，继发性闭经定义为无月经超过六个月。引起闭经的原因有很多，如核型为XY的女性的子宫缺如、处女膜闭锁引起的月经血无法流出、子宫内膜失调例如子宫瘢痕时的内膜缺如（Asherman综合征）、过早绝经时内膜萎缩或多囊卵巢综合征的激素紊乱。

原发性

原发性闭经已在青春期疾病中讲述。

继发性

继发性闭经最常见的原因是下丘脑抑制（图 40）、高催乳素血症（通常由催乳素瘤引起，图41）或多囊卵巢综合征。其他原因包括甲状腺疾病、肾上腺疾病、卵巢早衰与席汉综合征。席汉综合征是由于垂体前部产后缺血性坏死引发的垂体功能减退。妊娠期增生的腺垂体对低血压更为敏感，严重的产后出血会导致席汉综合征。

闭经、激素水平正常、有排卵的女性应怀疑其有Asherman综合征，尤其是曾做过某种形式子宫手术的妇女，如人流或刮宫术，这些手术会引起宫腔粘连。妊娠与自然绝经是生理性闭经。当女性主诉有继发性闭经时，应考虑是否存在妊娠与自然绝经。

Amenorrhoea

Amenorrhoea is defined as the failure to menstruate. It can be classified as primary (menstruation fails to start) or secondary, which is defined as the cessation of periods for more than 6 months. Amenorrhoea may be due to the absence of the uterus, as in an XY female, blockage of the outflow tract owing to an imperforate hymen, or endometrial disturbances, i.e. absence as in uterine scarring (Asherman syndrome), atrophy as in premature menopause, or hormonal imbalance as in polycystic ovarian syndrome.

Primary

Primary amenorrhoea has been mentioned in disorders of puberty (pg. 24).

Secondary

The most common causes of secondary amenorrhoea are hypothalamic suppression (Fig. 40), hyperprolactinaemia (usually due to a prolactinoma, Fig. 41) or polycystic ovarian syndrome. Other causes include thyroid disease, adrenal disease, premature ovarian failure and Sheehan syndrome. Sheehan syndrome is a form of hypopituitarism caused by post-partum ischaemic necrosis of the anterior pituitary. The hyperplastic pituitary gland in pregnancy is more susceptible to hypotension and severe post-partum haemorrhage may precipitate Sheehan syndrome.

Asherman syndrome should be suspected in women who have amenorrhoea and have normal hormonal profiles with evidence of ovulation, particularly in women who have had some form of uterine surgery, for example termination of pregnancy or dilatation and curettage (D&C), which could precipitate the formation of intrauterine adhesions. Pregnancy and natural menopause are physiological courses of amenorrhoea. When a woman presents with secondary amenorrhea pregnancy and natural menopause should always be considered.

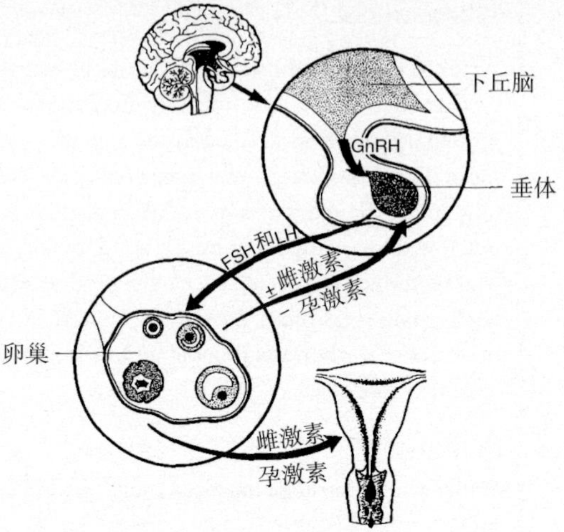

图 40 下丘脑 - 垂体 - 卵巢轴
Hypothalamic-pituitary-ovarian axis

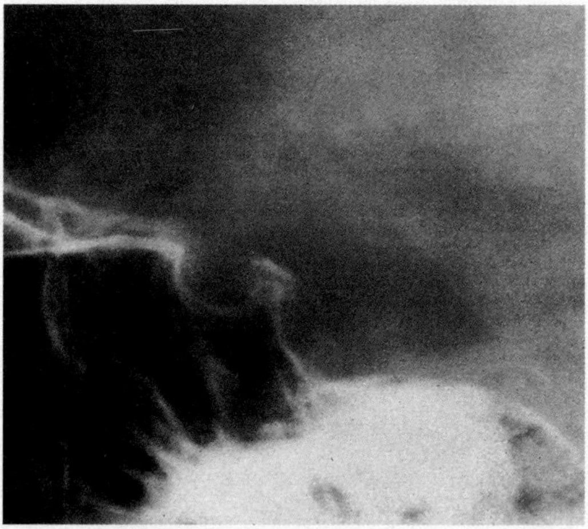

图 41 垂体窝增大的头部 X 线
Skull X-ray of enlarged pituitary fossa

功能失调性子宫出血

定义 排除盆腔疾病后确定的异常子宫出血。

病因 不清。

分类 分为无排卵性和排卵性两类。

临床特征 大多数患者有大量阴道规则或不规则流血。仅依靠病史很难精确评估流血量。可以通过收集所有止血棉塞和卫生垫以及应用碱性正铁血红素实验进行血液丢失定量的测定，但在临床很少采用。

腹部及盆腔的检查应未发现异常。

检查 为了排除盆腔疾病，必须进行彻底的盆腔检查，包括：宫颈涂片和经阴道超声（图 42），如有适应证还可行子宫内膜活检（图 43）。根据临床情况还可使用腹腔镜、宫腔镜（图 44）或彩色多普勒检查。

处理 *无排卵性功血*　青春期口服避孕药将使撤退性出血减少、月经规律并减少痛苦。围绝经期妇女适合应用激素替代治疗或周期孕激素疗法（排除子宫疾病后）。

排卵性功血　非甾体抗炎药、口服避孕药、达那唑和抗纤维蛋白溶解药或含孕激素节育系统（intrauterine system，IUS）是主要方法。如果上述方法均失败，可行内膜切除 / 消融或者子宫切除。

Dysfunctional uterine bleeding

Definition

Abnormal uterine bleeding after pelvic pathology has been excluded.

Aetiology

Not known.

Classification

Cases can be divided into anovulatory or ovulatory.

Clinical features

The majority of patients will report heavy bleeding, which may be regular or irregular. It is extremely difficult to make an accurate assessment of the amount of bleeding by relying on history alone. Quantitative measurement of blood loss can be made by collecting all the tampons and sanitary pads and using the alkalin haematin test but is rarely done in clinical practice.

On abdominal and pelvic examination there should be no abnormalities detected.

Investigations

To exclude pelvic pathology, a thorough pelvic assessment must be made including cervical smear, transvaginal ultrasound (Fig. 42), and endometrial biopsy (Fig. 43) if indicated. Laparoscopy, hysteroscopy (Fig. 44) or colour Doppler studies may be used, depending on the clinical situation.

Management

Anovulatory In adolescents the oral contraceptive pill will make the withdrawal bleeds lighter, regular and less painful. In the perimenopausal woman, hormone replacement therapy or cyclical progestogens (after exclusion of uterine pathology) would be appropriate.

Ovulatory Non-steroidal anti-inflammatory drugs, the oral contraceptive pill, danazol and antifibrinolytic drugs or the progesterone-releasing intrauterine system (IUS) are the main options. Endometrial resection/ablation or hysterectomy are used if the above measures fail.

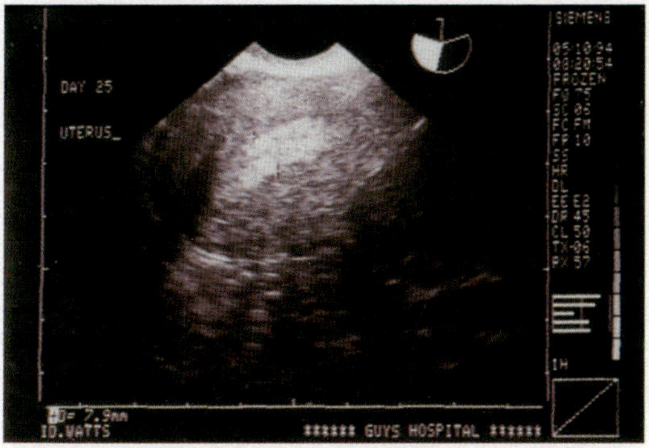

图 42　经阴道超声检查子宫内膜
Transvaginal ultrasound scan of endometrium

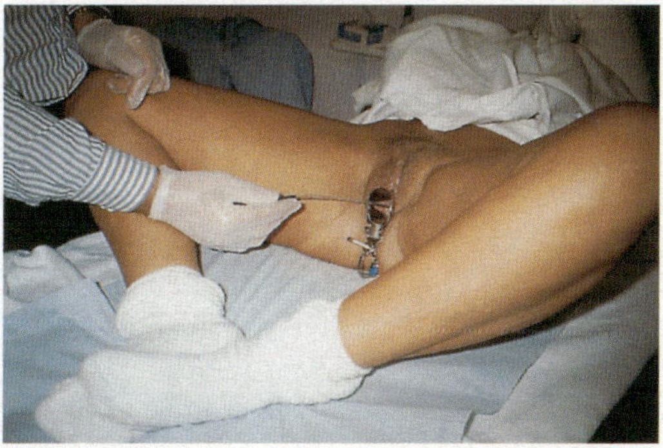

图 43　内膜活检
Endometrial biopsy

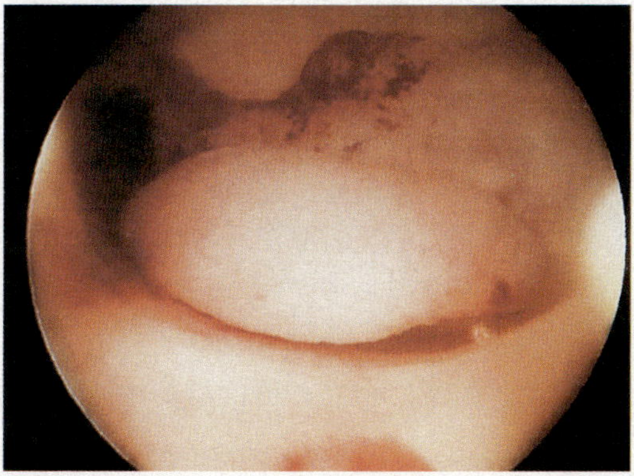

图 44　内膜息肉的宫腔镜图像
Hysteroscopic view of an endometrial polyp

“自然”方法

排卵期最易受孕：一个月经周期为28天的妇女，排卵大约发生在上次月经后的第14天左右。精液在生殖道存活可达到7天，所以为了避免怀孕应在排卵前一周停止性交，并建议持续到至少排卵后2天。排卵可以通过下列方法预测：

- 监测既往月经周期（节律法）
- 利用排卵时体温升高来确定“安全期”（图45）
- 判断宫颈黏液，它在排卵期变得量多而稀薄

这些方法的失败率高，每年100名妇女中有25例妊娠。

体外射精（射精前把阴茎从阴道中撤出）是广泛应用的避孕方法，但不是特别有效。

屏障避孕法

避孕套 含有杀精子剂如9-壬苯醇醚的避孕套是非常有效的，每年100名妇女中仅有2~3例失败。避孕套也作为性传播疾病的一种物理屏障，还可应用女性避孕套（图46）。

避孕帽 隔膜（图47）是应用最普遍的；其他类型包括宫颈和穹窿帽。当使用杀精药物时，隔膜与避孕套的效果是一样，并具有杀精作用。避孕帽由一个薄的圆顶橡胶乳粘在一个金属圆环上组成。查体后决定所需尺寸。它应该覆盖宫颈，隔膜的前缘在耻骨联合后，后缘在后穹窿。性交前插入，性交后至少六小时后取下。

其他方法 当前可用的还有浸有9-壬苯醇醚的一次性海绵，但它们价格昂贵并且不是很有效。

'Natural' methods

Highest fertility occurs at ovulation: in a 28-day cycle this occurs about 14 days after the last menstrual period. Sperm may survive in the genital tract for up to 7 days; therefore, to avoid conception, discontinue intercourse one week before ovulation is expected and recommence it not less than 2 days after ovulation has occurred. Ovulation may be predicted by:

- monitoring previous cycles (rhythm method)
- using the rise in body temperature with ovulation to determine the 'safe period' (Fig. 45)
- assessing the cervical mucus which becomes profuse and watery (*Spinbarkeit*) at ovulation.

The failure rates for these methods may be as high as 25 pregnancies per 100 women years.

Coitus interruptus (removal of the penis from the vagina before ejaculation) is a widely used method of contraception; not particularly effective.

Barrier methods

Condoms When used with a spermicide, e.g. Nonoxynol-9, condoms are effective, resulting in only 2-3 failures per 100 women years. Condoms also act as a physical barrier to the transmission of many sexually transmitted infections; female condoms are also available (Fig. 46).

Caps The diaphragm (Fig. 47) is the most commonly used; other types include cervical and vault caps. When used with spermicide, a diaphragm is as effective as a condom and spermicide. It consists of a thin latex rubber dome attached to a circular metal spring. The size required is determined during an examination. It should cover the cervix, with the anterior edge of the diaphragm lying behind the symphysis pubis and the posterior edge in the posterior fornix. It should be inserted prior to intercourse and should not be removed for at least 6 h afterwards.

Others Disposable sponges impregnated with Nonoxynol-9 are currently available, but they are expensive to buy and not very effective.

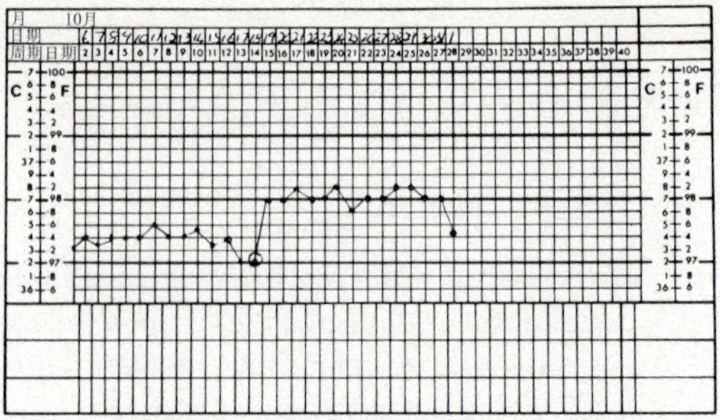

图 45 体温图——有排卵的双相型。排卵后体温上升并且持续到下次月经之前
Temperature chart — ovulatory biphasic pattern. Temperature rise follows ovulation and persists until just prior to menstruation

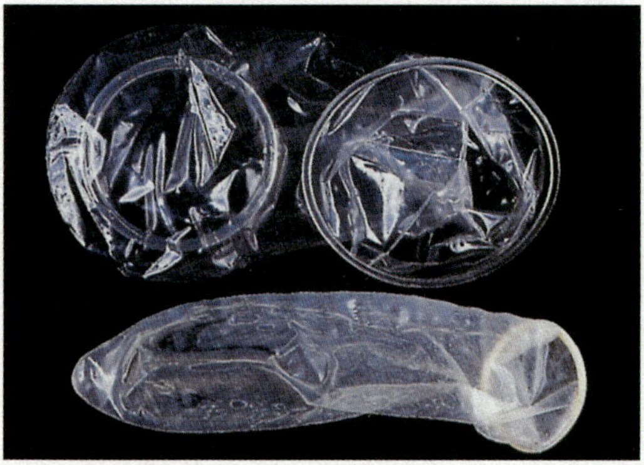

图 46 男用和女用避孕套
Male and female condoms

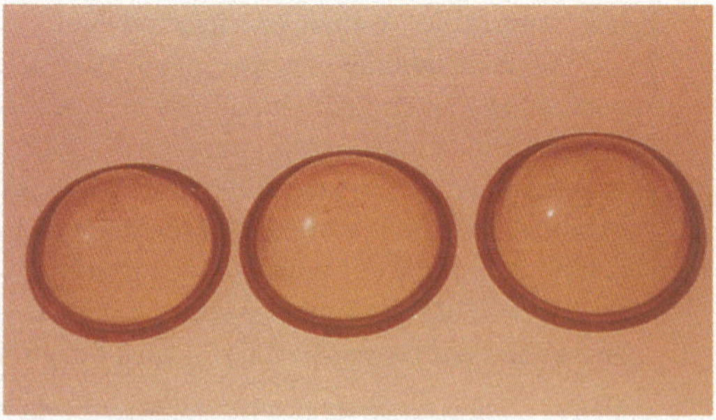

图 47 隔膜
Diaphragms

激素避孕法

复方口服避孕药物 包括雌激素和孕激素。每周期用药21天，停药7天，在停药期间出现药物撤退性出血。复方药物作用于下丘脑和垂体，通过负反馈引起对GnRH、FSH和LH的抑制，从而阻止排卵。子宫内膜也变得不适合受精卵着床。复方药物中的孕激素成分使得宫颈黏液不利于精子穿过，可能会干扰输卵管功能。这种复方药物禁用于激素依赖性肿瘤（乳腺、子宫内膜和滋养细胞）的妇女。血栓栓塞、动脉疾病、心脏瓣膜疾病、偏头痛、凝血功能障碍、肝疾病都是该药的禁忌证。吸烟、高血压、糖尿病是相对禁忌证。复方避孕药被认为是目前最有效的可逆性避孕措施（图 48）。

单纯孕激素药物 这类药不一定抑制排卵，其作用在子宫内膜、宫颈黏液和输卵管。单纯的孕激素药物应在每天同一时间服用，不应间断。服药后4 ~ 6小时对宫颈黏液的最大效果能够显现。即便是有很好的依从性，单纯孕激素药物还是不如复方药物有效。

己酸孕酮注射 应用足够大剂量，能够引起:

- 抑制排卵
- 使子宫内膜萎缩
- 使子宫黏液黏稠

这种避孕药有效、安全、方便，而且可逆，然而有些妇女会出现体重增加和阴道不规则流血。

皮下埋埴 每三年皮下埋置一杆依托孕烯（图49）。

Hormonal contraception

Combined oral contraceptive pills Contain both oestrogen and progesterone. They are taken cyclically for 21 days with a 7-day break. During the 'pill-free week', a withdrawal bleed is experienced. The combined pill acts on the hypothalamus and pituitary causing inhibition of GnRH, FSH and LH by negative feedback, thus preventing ovulation. The endometrium is also rendered unsuitable for implantation. The progesterone element of the combined pill makes the cervical mucus impenetrable to sperm and may also interfere with fallopian tube function. The combined pill should not be used by women with hormone-dependent tumours (breast, endometrium, trophoblast). Thromboembolism, arterial disease, valvular heart disease, focal migraine, clotting abnormalities and liver disease are all contraindications to pill usage. Smoking, hypertension and diabetes are considered 'relative contraindications'. The combined pill is the most effective reversible method of contraception currently available (Fig. 48).

Progesterone-only pills These do not necessarily inhibit ovulation; they act on the endometrium, the endocervical mucus and the fallopian tubes. Progesterone-only preparations should be taken at the same time every day, without any breaks. The maximal effect on cervical mucus is seen 4~6 h after taking the pills. Even with good compliance, progesterone-only pills are less effective than combined pills.

Depot progestogen injections Used in sufficiently high doses, these will:

- inhibit ovulation
- render the endometrium atrophic
- thicken the cervical mucus

This form of contraception is effective, safe, convenient and reversible. Some women will, however, suffer from weight gain and bleeding irregularities.

Implants One rod of etonogestrel is inserted subdermally every 3 years (Fig. 49).

Pearl索引是用来计算避孕方法的有效率，定义如下：如果100名妇女按照指导应用合适的避孕方法，一年内这些妇女中的怀孕的妇女数量（或者是应用避孕方法的一年内出现不需要妊娠的妇女百分比）。这与来自“典型应用”的实际失败率截然不同，更不是该方法的“完美应用”。

不避孕	80 ~ 90	避孕贴	< 1
男性避孕套	2	宫内节育器	1 ~ 2
女性避孕套	5	LNG-IUS	1
隔膜与避孕帽	4 ~ 8	自然家庭计划	2 ~ 6
COCP	< 1	人格	6
POP	1	女性绝育	0.5
可注射的孕激素	< 1	男性绝育	0.05
孕激素埋植	< 1		

图 48　Pearl 索引
The Pearl Index

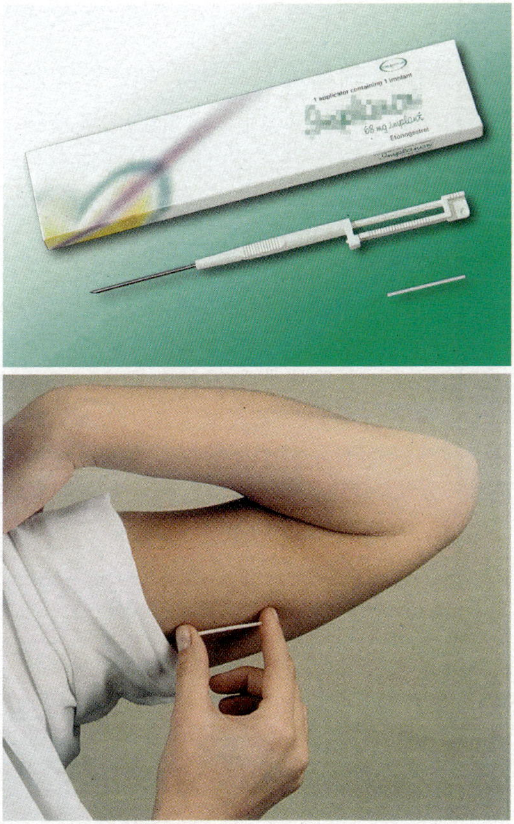

图 49　孕激素埋植
Progesterone implant

紧急避孕 共两片药，每片含有750mg的左旋-18-甲基炔诺孕酮。第一片药在无防护性性生活后的72小时内服用，第二片药相隔12小时后服用。这种方法防止 86% 的预期怀孕，副反应可能出现恶心。

宫内节育器（intrauterine contraceptive devices，IUCD）

宫内节育器（图50）由医生采用无菌技术放置入宫腔。通过改变 / 抑制精子移动和卵子运输起作用。对异物的无菌性炎症反应使胚泡着床受阻。它是一种安全、高效以及可逆的避孕措施。但它必须由医师安放，并且需要随访。有盆腔炎、宫内妊娠或子宫畸形的妇女不应该安放节育器。它也可以用于紧急避孕。在无防护性性生活的 5 天之内安放有效。

释放孕激素的宫内系统（intrauterine system, IUS）

孕激素释放到宫腔内，抑制内膜增殖，使宫颈黏液黏稠。这一方法还可减少月经血量和减轻痛经。它也是最有效的可逆避孕措施之一。

绝育术

女性绝育术是输卵管阻断。可以通过腹腔镜下切除，用夹子、环闭塞输卵管或者电凝输卵管，或做小切口开腹手术行输卵管阻断（图 51）。此方法高效但不可逆，失败率大约为 0.1%。

男性绝育术是女性绝育术的一个好的替代方法，当夫妻就诊于妇科门诊要求行绝育术时应当与夫妻双方共同商讨。

Postcoital contraception Two tablets each containing 750mg of levonorgestrel. The first tablet must be taken within 72h of unprotected intercourse and the second 12h later. This regimen prevented 86% of expected pregnancies. Nausea may be experienced as a side effect.

Intrauterine contraceptive devices (IUCD)

The IUCD (Fig. 50) is placed in the uterus by a doctor using a sterile technique. It acts by altering/inhibiting sperm migration and ovum transport. The sterile inflammatory response to the presence of a foreign body inhibits implantation of the blastocyst. It is a safe, highly effective and reversible form of contraception, but it must be fitted by a doctor and requires follow-up care. An IUCD should not be fitted in women who have had pelvic inflammatory disease, or if there is an intrauterine pregnancy or uterine abnormality. It can be used as a method of postcoital contraception. To be effective if must be fitted within 5 days of unprotected intercourse.

Progesterone releasing intrauterine system (IUS)

Progestogens are released into the uterine cavity and prevent proliferation and cause thickening of the cervical mucus. The devices also reduce menstrual blood loss and dysmenorrhoea. They are one of the most effective reversible methods of contraception.

Sterilization

Female methods of sterilization involve the blockage of the fallopian tubes. This can be achieved by excision or occlusion with clips (Fig. 51), rings, or by diathermy via the laparoscope or a mini-laparotomy. It is highly effective and should be considered irreversible. The failure rate is about 0.1%.

Male sterilization is a good alternative to female sterilization and should be discussed with couples presenting to the gynaecology clinic requesting sterilization.

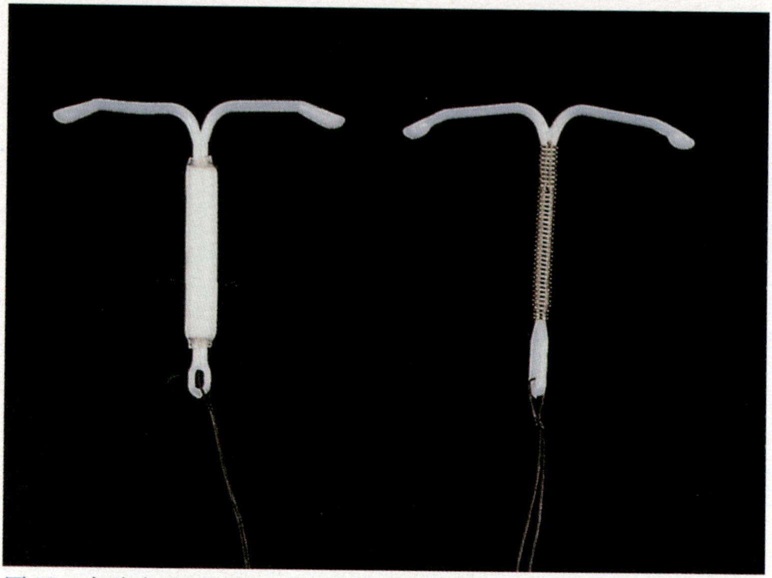

图 50　宫腔内避孕装置：（左）含有孕激素的宫内节育器；（右）Nova T 型宫内节育器
Intrauterine contraceptive devices: (left) Progestagen-containing IUS; (right) Nova T IUCD

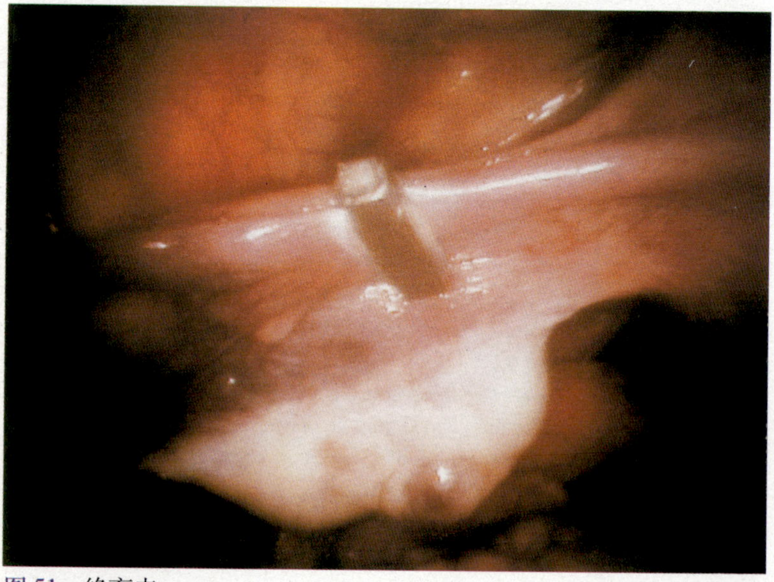

图 51　绝育夹
Sterilization clip

流产

定义

在妊娠 24 周前自发的妊娠终止。

发病率

流产的发生率占全部妊娠的 15% ~ 25%。

分类

流产可分为以下几种（图 52）：

- *先兆流产*：胚胎仍存活，宫口未开。
- *难免流产*：胚胎可能还存活，但宫口已开。
- *不全流产*：妊娠产物已部分排出体外。
- *完全流产*：胚胎和胎盘已全部排出体外。
- *稽留流产*：胚胎已死亡但尚未排出体外。

病因

大多数流产是由于染色体缺陷。如流产发生在妊娠前三个月内则没有必要检查，除非该妇女已经连续经历三次自然流产。病因有以下几方面：

- 异常孕体（染色体或结构的异常）
- 免疫因素
- 子宫畸形
- 宫颈机能不全
- 内分泌因素
- 母体疾病（包括系统性红斑狼疮）
- 感染
- 毒素和细胞毒性药物
- 外伤

Miscarriage

Definition

A spontaneous loss of pregnancy before 24 weeks.

Incidence

15%~25% of all pregnancies end in miscarriage.

Classification

Miscarriage can be classified as follows (Fig. 52):

- *Threatened miscarriage*: fetus is still viable, and the cervical os is closed.
- *Inevitable miscarriage*: fetus may still be alive but the cervical os is open.
- *Incomplete miscarriage*: some products of conception have been expelled already.
- *Complete miscarriage*: fetus and placental tissue have all been expelled.
- *Delayed miscarriage*: the pregnancy has succumbed but has not been expelled (Fig. 52).

Aetiology

The majority of miscarriages are due to chromosomal defects. If they are in the first trimester it is not necessarily helpful investigating women who miscarry - unless they have had three consecutive spontaneous miscarriages. The causes can be:

- abnormal conceptus (chromosomal or structural)
- immunological
- uterine abnormality
- cervical incompetence
- endocrine
- maternal disease (including systemic lupus erythematosus)
- infection
- toxins and cytotoxic drugs
- trauma.

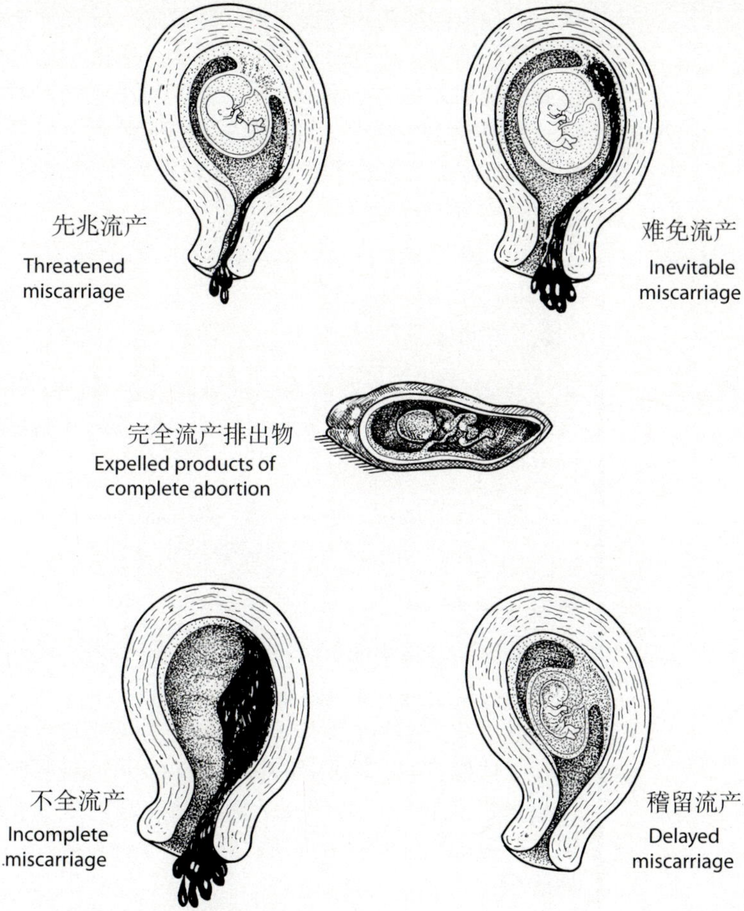

图 52 流产分类的图形表示
Diagrammatic representation of types of miscarriage

临床特点

病人出现停经后阴道流血。可伴随腹痛。妊娠症状可能已经消失。检查时可有下腹压痛。阴道出血量可由点滴到大量流血不等。子宫大小可小于妊娠周数（如妊娠物已排出）、与妊娠周数相符或大于妊娠周数（如发生宫腔内积血）。根据流产的不同时期，宫颈口可关闭或开放。

鉴别诊断

- 异位妊娠
- 葡萄胎
- 功能失调性子宫出血

检查

如果宫颈口已开，妊娠无法继续，无须进一步检查。如果宫颈口未开，超声可鉴定宫腔内的胚胎是否可存活（图 53）。

治疗

先兆流产没有确切的治疗方法。难免流产、不全流产、完全流产和稽留流产都需要清宫（图 54）。

复发性流产

越来越多的证据表明复发性流产的妇女有抗心磷脂抗体和抗磷脂抗体（抗磷脂抗体综合征）。有三次或三次以上流产史的妇女应该选择一个专业机构以便进行上述检查。抗磷脂抗体综合征妇女可有妊娠晚期疾病的风险，包括先兆子痫和胎儿宫内生长受限。一旦确定胚胎存活即使用肝素和小剂量阿司匹林治疗。

Clinical features

Patients will present with amenorrhoea followed by vaginal bleeding. Pain may be present. The symptoms of pregnancy may have disappeared. On examination there may be lower abdominal tenderness. The bleeding may vary from spotting to heavy bleeding. The uterine size may be smaller than dates (if products have been expelled), the same size, or larger than dates (if bleeding has occurred into the uterine cavity). The cervix may be closed or open depending on the stage of the miscarriage.

Differential diagnosis

- Ectopic pregnancy
- Hydatidiform mole
- Dysfunctional uterine bleeding

Investigations

If the cervical os is open, the pregnancy will not continue and no further investigations are needed. If the os is closed, an ultrasound scan will determine whether a viable fetus is present in the uterine cavity (Fig. 53).

Management

There is no proven treatment for a threatened abortion. Inevitable, incomplete, complete and missed abortions all require evacuation of the uterus (Fig. 54).

Recurrent miscarriage

There is increasing evidence that women who recurrently miscarry may have anticardiolipin and antiphospholipid antibodies (antiphospholipid antibody syndrome). Women who have three or more miscarriages should be referred to a specialist unit where this can be investigated. Women with antiphospholipid antibody syndrome also appear to be at risk of later pregnancy problems including pre-eclampsia and intrauterine growth restriction. The treatment may include heparin and the use of low-dose aspirin from as soon as a viable pregnancy is diagnosed.

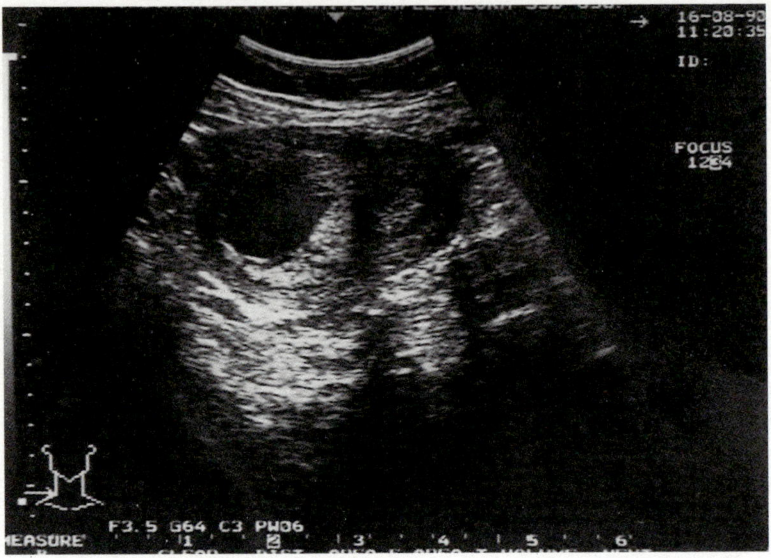

图 53　双角子宫稽留流产的超声图像
Ultrasound picture of a delayed miscarriage in a bicornuate uterus

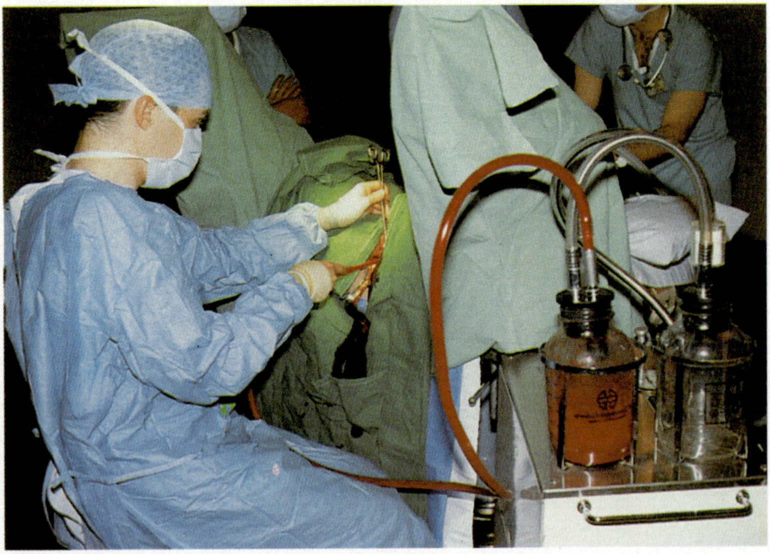

图 54　清宫术
Surgical evacuation of the uterus

异位妊娠：诊断

定义	受精卵着床于子宫腔之外（大多在输卵管壶腹部）。
病因	阻碍受精卵在输卵管中运行的任何因素都可导致异位妊娠。最常见的原因是既往盆腔感染。
病理生理学	受精卵沿输卵管运行延缓并着床于输卵管黏膜，对输卵管壁的侵蚀和扩张导致输卵管内或腹膜内出血(图55)。子宫内膜受到滋养层分泌的激素刺激发生蜕膜反应。
临床特点	症状 典型症状是停经后不规则点滴出血或阴道流血和一侧（也可为双侧）腹部疼痛。 体征 依据输卵管是否破裂，体征有所不同。如有输卵管破裂，病人可出现休克。 腹部体征可表现为一侧下腹压痛和反跳痛，甚至有板状腹。内诊常常有宫颈刺激症和一侧压痛，并可在一侧扪及包块。
鉴别诊断	• 流产 • 盆腔感染

Ectopic pregnancy: diagnosis

Definition

The implantation of a pregnancy outside the uterine cavity (usually in the ampullary part of the fallopian tube).

Aetiology

Any factor that will decrease embryo transport along the tube can lead to an ectopic pregnancy. The most common cause is previous pelvic infection.

Patho-physiology

The fertilized ovum is delayed in its transport along the tube and implants on the tubal mucosa. Intratubal or intraperitoneal bleeding occurs as a result of erosion and distension of the tubal wall (Fig. 55). The uterine endometrium undergoes decidualization in response to the hormonal stimulus of the trophoblast.

Clinical features

Symptoms

Classically, the patient will have had amenorrhoea followed by irregular spotting or vaginal bleeding and unilateral pain (may be bilateral).

Signs

These will vary depending on whether tubal rupture has occurred. If tubal rupture has occurred the patient may be in shock.
The abdominal signs can vary from unilateral lower abdominal tenderness with rebound to a rigid abdomen with guarding. Vaginally there is usually cervical excitation, unilateral tenderness, and a mass may be felt on one side.

Differential diagnosis

- Miscarriage
- Pelvic infection

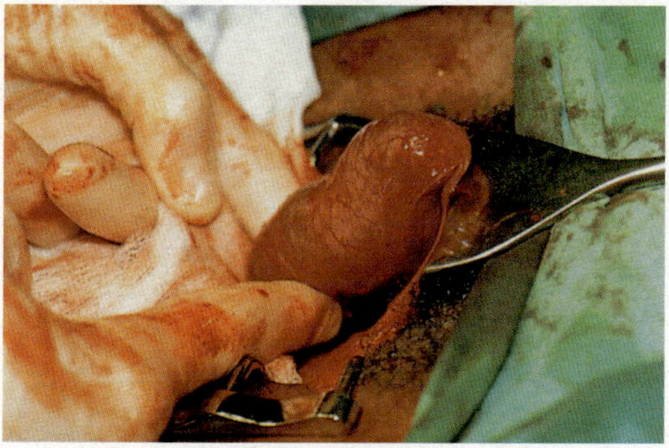

图 55　异位妊娠扩张输卵管
Ectopic gestation distending the fallopian tube

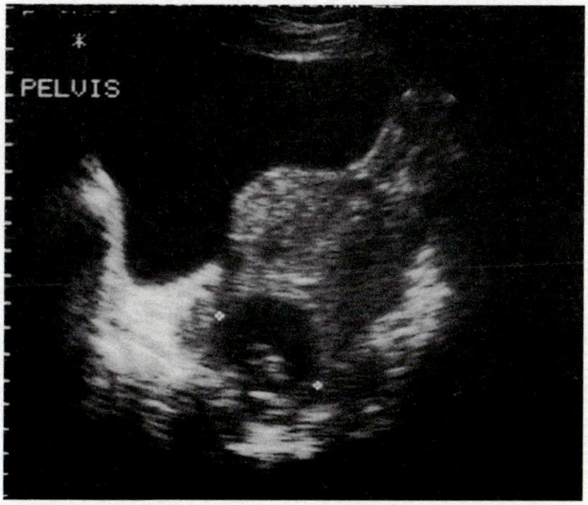

图 56　妊娠囊位于宫旁，使膀胱成锯齿状
Gestation sac lateral to the uterus that is indenting the bladder

异位妊娠：治疗

检查

超声 有助于鉴别宫内妊娠或在宫腔外的异位妊娠（图 56）。并且在直肠子宫陷凹可见游离积液。

血标本 定量检测 HCG、FBC 和交叉配血。

治疗

综合 HCG 定量、超声检查和临床特点决定保守治疗还是介入治疗。如果 HCG 水平未降至满意水平或临床症状未消退，则可采用腹腔镜。

腹腔镜 输卵管表现为扩张或充血（图 57），盆腔中也可以有游离液体。如对侧输卵管正常，可选择腹腔镜输卵管切除术。

开腹手术 适于异位妊娠破裂导致休克者或使用腹腔镜不安全者。

少数患者可发生输卵管流产，胚胎可种植在腹腔内（图 58）。

预后

手术后宫腔内妊娠率 50%，再次宫外孕发生率 20%。

仅 1/3 的妇女可妊娠至足月。

Ectopic pregnancy: Management

Investigations

Ultrasound scan is useful to confirm an intrauterine pregnancy, or an ectopic pregnancy can be seen outside the uterine cavity (see Fig. 56), and free fluid can be seen in the pouch of Douglas.

Blood sampling Quantitative HCG assay and FBC, and cross-matching.

Management

The quantitative HCG, the ultrasound findings and the clinical picture will determine whether conservative or interventional management is appropriate. If the level of HCG does not fall at an acceptable rate and/or the clinical situation is not resolving, then laparoscopy is mandatory.

Laparoscopy The fallopian tube may appear distended or filled with blood (Fig. 57) and/or there may be free blood in the pelvis. Laparoscopic salpingectomy (removal of the tube) is the treatment of choice if the other tube is laparoscopically normal.

Laparotomy Should be considered if the patient is in shock due to a ruptured ectopic pregnancy or any situation that can not be safely dealt with laparoscopically.

Occasionally a tubal abortion may have occurred and the fetus may be free in the peritoneal cavity (Fig. 58).

Prognosis

The intrauterine pregnancy rate after surgery is 50% and the repeat ectopic rate is 20%.

Only one-third of women will proceed to have a successful term baby.

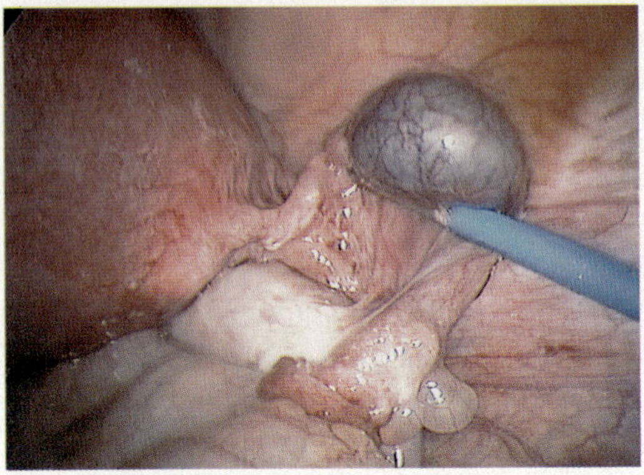

图 57 腹腔镜下充血膨胀的输卵管
Fallopian tube distended with blood as seen laparoscopically

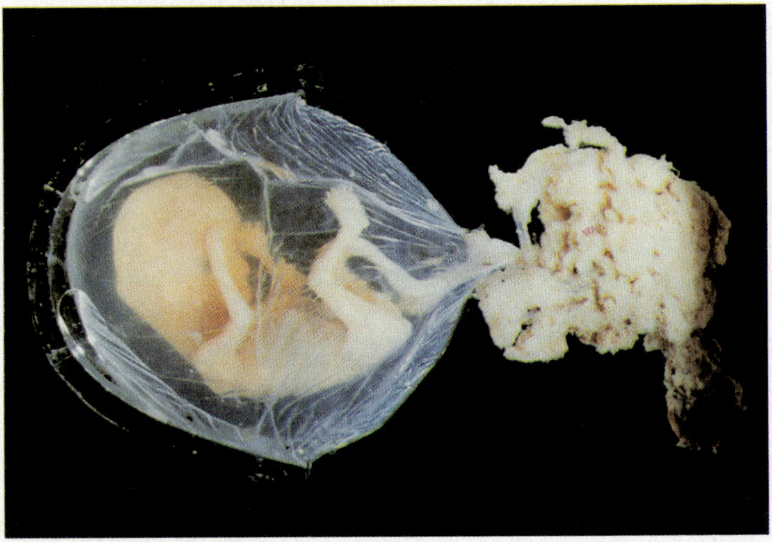

图 58 腹腔内游离胚胎
Fetus found free in the peritoneal cavity

滋养细胞疾病

定义 葡萄胎是一种滋养细胞肿瘤。

发病率 从地域分布看，亚洲国家发病率明显高于西方国家。

病因 不明确。

分类 *完全性葡萄胎* 无胚胎。染色体核型均来自父系，有 46 条染色体。

部分性葡萄胎 有胚胎。有69条染色体，一套多余的染色体来自父系。

侵袭性葡萄胎 可浸润子宫和/或转移至肺。

临床特点 症状通常为妊娠期前3个月阴道不规则流血。子宫可大于相应妊娠周数。无胎心搏动，先兆子痫可能发生早，可能有卵巢黄素化囊肿。

检查 超声显示“落雪征”，且无胚胎（图59）。β-HCG水平很高。应做X线胸片以排除肺转移。

处理 吸净宫腔内水泡状囊泡（图60）。如果子宫体积过大，可羊膜腔外应用前列腺素。年龄较大的妇女可行子宫切除术。确保所有患者的β-HCG水平降至正常是随访的重点。

随访

随访期限通过英国的两个中心协调确定。如果患者在清宫后56天内HCG水平降至正常，随访限于6个月。在此期间患者应避孕。如果HCG在清宫后8周未降至正常，需随访2年。

预后 1/30的葡萄胎可发展为恶性的滋养细胞肿瘤即绒膜癌。化疗是主要的治疗手段，密切随访是必要的。

下次妊娠时必须尽早通过超声检查排除葡萄胎，并且在分娩后3周需做HCG检查。

Trophoblastic disease

Definition Hydatidiform mole is a tumour of trophoblast.

Incidence Varies geographically, with a higher incidence in Asiatic countries than in the West.

Aetiology Unknown.

Classification *Complete mole* No fetus is present and the chromosomal complement is totally paternal. There are 46 chromosomes.

Partial mole Fetus is present. There are 69 chromosomes and the extra set is of paternal origin.

Invasive mole May penetrate the uterus and/or metastasize to the lungs.

Clinical features The symptoms are usually irregular bleeding in the first trimester of pregnancy. The uterus may be larger than dates and the fetal heart is usually absent. Pre-eclampsia may develop early, and theca lutein cysts may be palpable.

Investigations Ultrasound will demonstrate a 'snowstorm' appearance, and the fetus will not be seen (Fig. 59). Beta-HCG level is very high. A chest X-ray should be done to exclude pulmonary metastases.

Management Suction evacuation of the hydropic vesicles (Fig. 60). If uterine size is too large, extra-amniotic prostaglandins are used. Hysterectomy may be done in the older woman. It is essential to follow all women to ensure that the beta-HCG levels disappear.

Follow-up

This is co-ordinated through two centres in the UK. If the patient's HCG level reaches the normal range within 56 days of evacuation, follow-up is limited to 6 months, during which time the patients are advised not to conceive. If the HCG has not returned to normal within 8 weeks of evacuation, follow-up is for 2 years.

Prognosis One in 30 moles develops into choriocarcinoma-a malignant tumour of trophoblastic tissue. Chemotherapy is the mainstay of treatment and close follow-up is essential.

In subsequent pregnancies women must attend early to exclude molar pregnancy by ultrasound and an HCG should be performed 3 weeks after delivery.

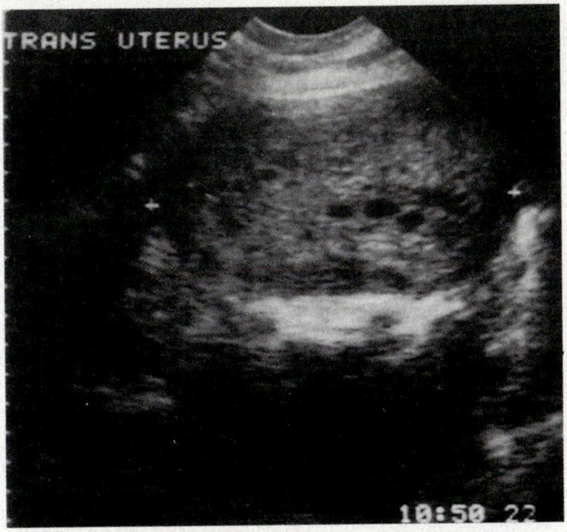

图 59　葡萄胎的超声图像
Ultrasound picture of hydatidiform mole

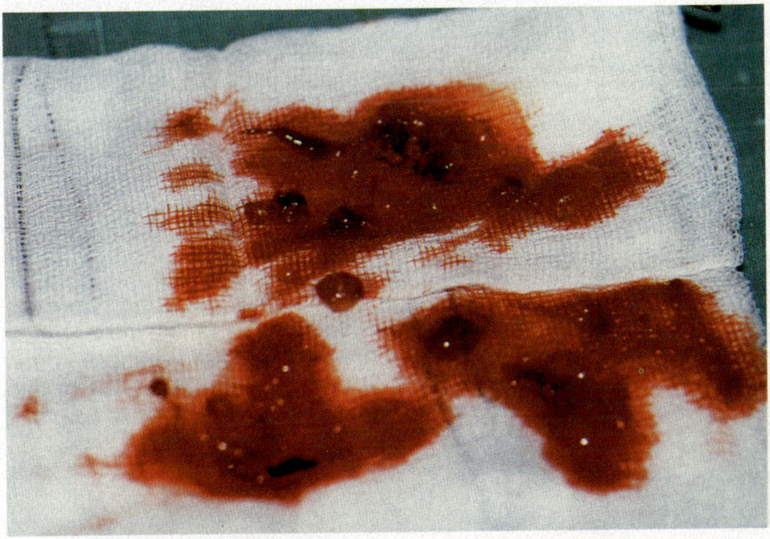

图 60　葡萄胎的水肿囊泡
Hydropic vesicles of hydatidiform mole

7 治疗性流产

定义 妊娠 24 周前人工终止妊娠。

分类 终止妊娠可能因为胚胎或母体因素。大多数因为继续妊娠可危害妇女的身体或精神健康。

检查 如果疑为妊娠，应行超声检查。如有需要可行全血细胞计数、血型、Rh 血型和血红蛋白电泳检查。

处理 终止妊娠时必需咨询。需两名职业医生填写适当的表格（图 61）。终止妊娠的方法依据妊娠时期。

孕激素拮抗剂 在妊娠 9 周前可选用孕激素拮抗剂，与前列腺素栓剂联合应用，导致“医学”上对妊娠的终止。

扩张宫颈和清宫术 扩张宫颈（如术前应用前列腺素栓剂可使手术更容易），然后清除子宫内容物，通常妊娠大于 14 周时需负压吸引。

前列腺素 在怀孕14周之后，需用前列腺素引产。可阴道内给药、羊膜腔内或羊膜腔外给药。无论哪一种方法，须行清宫术以确保宫腔被清空。米非司酮配伍米索前列醇越来越普遍。

Therapeutic abortion

Definition

Medical termination of pregnancy prior to 24 weeks' gestation.

Classification

Terminations can be performed for fetal or maternal reasons. Most are performed because the continuation of the pregnancy will cause risk to the physical or mental health of the woman.

Investigations

If gestation is in doubt, an ultrasound scan should be performed. Full blood count, blood group, Rhesus status and haemoglobin electrophoresis should be undertaken if indicated.

Management

Counselling is essential in pregnancy termination. The appropriate forms (Fig. 61) must be filled out with two certifying practitioners. The method of termination will depend on the gestation.

Progesterone antagonists These are used in combination with a prostaglandin pessary prior to 9 weeks' gestation, leading to a 'medical' termination of pregnancy.

Dilatation and evacuation The cervix is dilated (this can be made easier if a prostaglandin pessary is used prior to surgery) and then the uterine contents are removed, usually with a suction curettage (up to 14 weeks' gestation).

Prostaglandins Labour is induced with prostaglandins after 14 weeks' gestation. They can be administered as vaginal pessaries, intra-amniotically or extra-amniotically. Whatever the route, the procedure is followed by an evacuation of the uterus to ensure that the uterine cavity is empty. Mifepristone and gemeprost are becoming more popular.

可信　　　　流产通知

Please leave blank

1967 年流产法案

通知表（英格兰和威尔士）

本表由终止妊娠的操作者填写，7 天内用密封的信封寄至：

The Chief Medical Officer
Department of Health
Richmond House
79 Whitehall
LONDON
SW1A 2NS

或

The Chief Medical Officer
Welsh Office
Cathays Park
CARDIFF
CF1 3NQ

遵照威尔士的
终止妊娠的规定

请用大写字母填写，日期用数字填写

1. 终止妊娠操作者

姓名 ……………………

长期住址 ……………………

顺便提示，被终止妊娠的妇女姓名在背面，据我所知，本表格所填写的信息均正确。我进一步声明我在此之前参与 / 没有参与[†]提供证明 A，已经看过 / 没有看过和检查过 / 没有检查[†]过她。

签名 …………………… 日期 ……………………

2. 证明　在所有非急诊病例中，参与操作的操作者提供证明 A。

	1.在所有病例中将被完成	2.如果操作者提供证明 A 将不能完成
姓名	……………………	……………………
长期住址	……………………	……………………
	……………………	……………………

（在合适的框内打钩）

操作者 1 在提供证明前证明他看到 / 检查过孕妇吗？ ☐ 是 ☐ 否

操作者 2 在提供证明前证明他看到 / 检查过孕妇吗？ ☐ 是 ☐ 否

第 20 部分如有申请，不要完成填写　　　　请不要填这些框

3. 终止妊娠的地点名称和地址 ……………………

……………………

病人是否参加了英国国民健康保险，在相应机构同意地点终止妊娠？（在合适的框内打钩） ☐ 是 ☐ 否

[†]如果合适就去掉

从 HSA4（1991 年修正）

图 61　黄色表格（Crown 版权。经允许复制）
'Yellow form'. (Crown copyright. Reproduced by permission.)

低位生殖道感染

最常见表现是阴道分泌物增多和外阴阴道炎。

念珠菌

病因 大多病例的病因为白色念珠菌（一种类似酵母的真菌）。酵母菌存在阴道内而不引起症状。念珠菌不需要通过性传播，它可由肛门传播至外阴和阴道。一旦形成，它可通过无症状的性伴侣性交传播。

临床特征 酵母菌是引起阴道炎和阴道分泌物的原因。分泌物是特有的白色、颗粒状、无异味和刺激性。外阴可发红、水肿，和/或被覆白色分泌物（图62）。阴道里干酪样白带附着于阴道壁（图 63），可通过显微镜和高位阴道拭子革兰染色或适当培养基培养确定酵母菌。

治疗 治疗包括局部应用抗真菌药物、栓剂或膏剂。严重的病例需要系统治疗，应用口服抗真菌药如氟康唑。

阴道毛滴虫（Trichomonas vaginalis，TV）

病因 阴道毛滴虫寄生于阴道、尿道（男女均可）和上生殖道。它占引起阴道异常分泌物常见原因的第二位。它通过性传播，常与淋病有关。阴道分泌物是稀薄、黄色、有刺激性，通常为有异味的泡沫状分泌物，可引起阴道黏膜和宫颈充血（图 64）。可在阴道分泌物内加入一滴生理盐水并经显微镜确定病原菌。

8 Gynaecological infections

Lower genital tract infections

The most common manifestations are vaginal discharge and vulvovaginitis.

Candida (thrush)

Aetiology

Most cases are due to Candida albicans (a yeast-like fungus). Yeasts may be present in the vagina without causing symptoms. Candida is not necessarily sexually transmitted, it can spread from the anus to the vulva and vagina. Once established, however, it can be transmitted sexually even by an asymptomatic partner.

Clinical features

Yeasts are the most common cause of vaginitis and vaginal discharge. The discharge is characteristically white, particulate, non-offensive and irritant. The vulva may appear red and oedematous and/or covered in white discharge (Fig. 62). In the vagina, white discharge (the texture of cottage cheese) adheres to the vaginal walls (Fig. 63). Yeasts can be identified by microscopy and Gram staining of a high vaginal swab, and by culture in the appropriate medium.

Management

Treatment includes topical antifungal agents, pessaries and creams. Severe cases may require systemic therapy with oral antifungal agents, e.g. fluconazole.

Trichomonas vaginalis (TV)

Aetiology

TV is a flagellate parasite found in the vagina, the urethra (of both men and women) and in the upper genital tract. It is the second most common cause of vaginal discharge. It is sexually acquired and is often found in association with gonorrhoea. The vaginal discharge is thin, yellow, offensive and irritant, often appearing frothy and causing reddening of the vaginal epithelium and the cervix (see Fig. 64). The organism is identified by microscopy of a high vaginal sample mixed with a drop of saline.

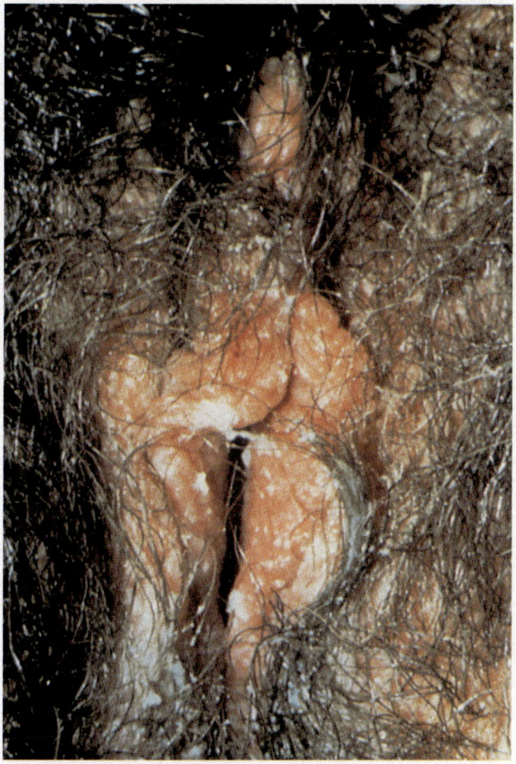

图 62　外阴假丝酵母病
Vulval candidiasis

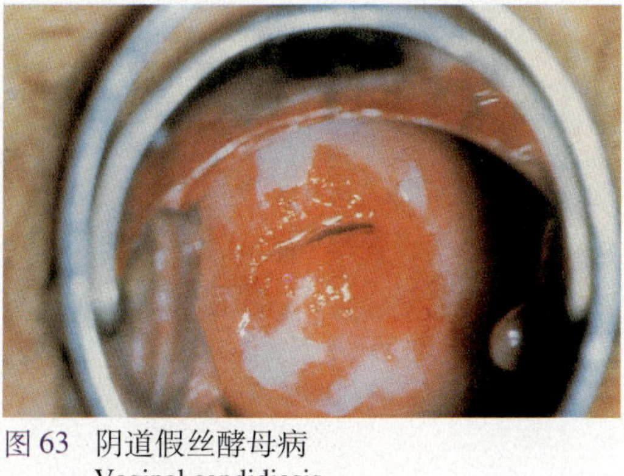

图 63　阴道假丝酵母病
Vaginal candidiasis

细菌性阴道病

它的特征为有异味的阴道分泌物，氨试验阳性，pH明显大于5，通过革兰染色涂片可见线索细胞。它是一种混合感染，包括阴道加德纳菌、厌氧菌（拟杆菌和消化链球菌）。

治疗为口服甲硝唑或克林霉素膏。其他原因也可引起阴道分泌物增多但分泌物正常，如排卵期、性兴奋或妊娠期。分泌物不正常可由化学刺激、异物刺激或退化性疾病引起。

疣（人类乳头状瘤病毒：HPV）

概述

疣是由人类乳头状瘤病毒引发。它可以是扁平状，肉眼无法见到，也可以是较大的外生性病灶。宫颈（图65）、阴道和外阴表面（图66）易感染。HPV是宫颈肿瘤生成的致病因素。潜伏期是3周至8个月。它表现为无痛性、慢速生长的外阴阴道肿物。鉴别诊断包括传染性软疣（由疱疹病毒引起）、湿疣（二期梅毒病损）和其他皮赘、痣或皮脂腺囊肿。

处理

以下治疗均可以：黄色树脂剂（一种细胞毒性制剂）、三氯醋酸、电烧、冷冻、切除。顽固性大面积的疣选用后三种方法。使用避孕套避孕。

Bacterial vaginosis

This is characterized by an offensive vaginal discharge that gives a positive amine test, has a pH greater than 5, and 'clue cells' seen on microscopy of a Gram stained smear. The cause is a mixed infection with *Gardnerella vaginalis* and anaerobic organisms including *Bacteroides species* and Peptostreptococcus.

Treatment is with oral metronidazole or clindamycin cream. Other causes of vaginal discharge include increased but normal vaginal secretion, e.g. at ovulation, during sexual excitement or during pregnancy, and abnormal discharge due to chemical irritants, foreign bodies or degenerative conditions.

Warts (human papilloma virus: HPV)

Description

Warts are caused by the human papilloma virus. They can be flat and undetectable to the naked eye, or large exophytic lesions. The cervix (Fig. 65), vaginal and vulval surfaces (Fig. 66) are all susceptible to infection. HPV has been strongly implicated as a causative factor in cervical neoplasia. The incubation period varies from 3 weeks to 8 months. It may present as painless slow-growing vulvovaginal lumps. The differential diagnoses include molluscum contagiosum (caused by a pox virus) condylomata lata (lesions of secondary syphylis) and other skin tags, naevi or sebaceous cysts.

Management

The following treatments are available: podophyllin (a cytotoxic agent), trichloracetic acid, electrocautery, cryocautery and excision. The last three are reserved for resistant and extensive warts. Barrier contraception is advised.

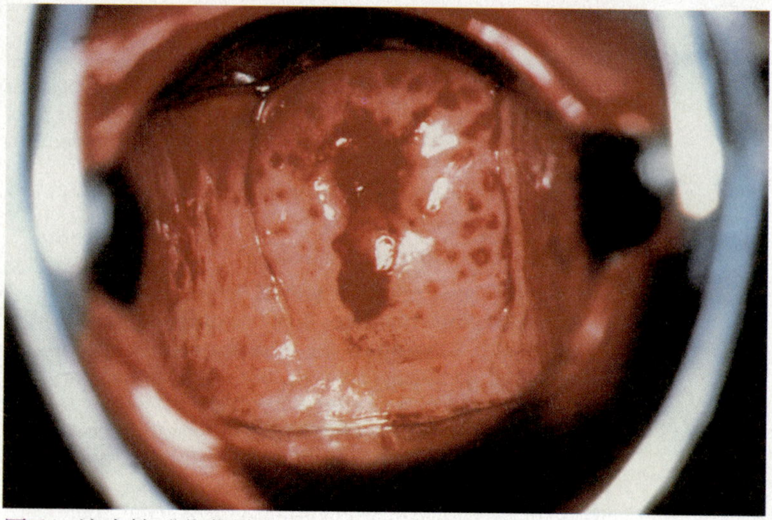

图 64　滴虫性“草莓样宫颈”
Trichomonal 'strawberry cervix'

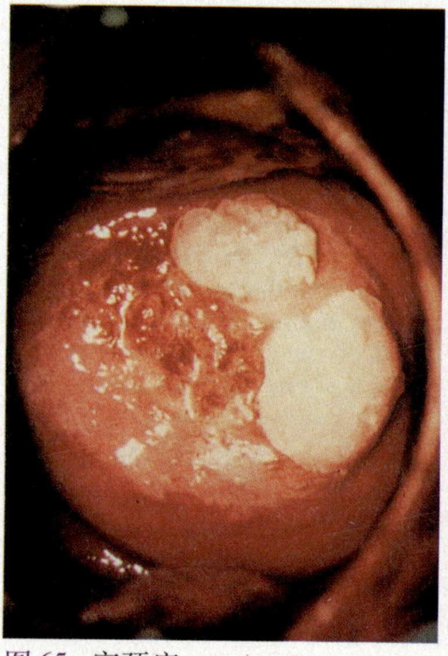

图 65　宫颈疣
Cervical warts

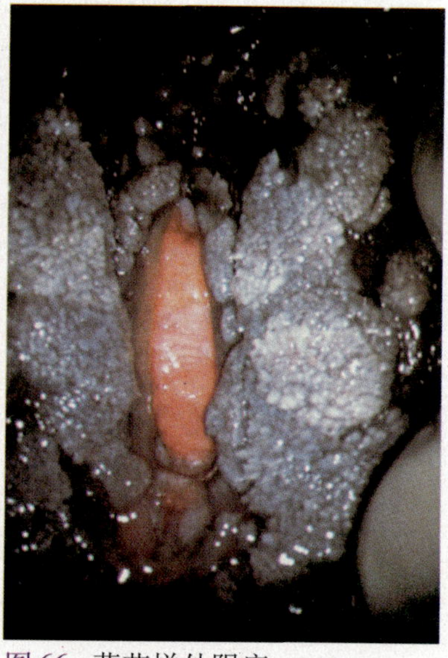

图 66　菜花样外阴疣
Florid vulval warts

单纯疱疹病毒（HSV）

病因

生殖器和肛门疱疹通常由Ⅱ型单纯疱疹病毒引起。而Ⅰ型单纯疱疹病毒通常引发口唇疱疹，也可引起生殖器感染。在英国，生殖器疱疹是生殖器溃疡最常见的原因。

临床特征

原发感染表现为前驱不适症状，继而出现水泡（图67）、溃疡、腹股沟淋巴结病，伴不适、发热及尿潴留。在女性，水泡好发于外阴（图68）、阴道和宫颈。原发感染的病变经过几周愈合，继发感染很常见。复发很常见，因为病毒在两次复发间期在节后神经根处潜伏。重复感染并不明显。诊断依据临床检查和溃疡的病毒培养。

处理

在初次发作时阿昔洛韦可减轻症状和病毒脱落的时间。除非连续治疗，否则阿昔洛韦不能阻止复发。

并发症

原发感染可引起全身并发症，包括肝炎、脊髓炎、脑炎、脑膜炎。在妊娠早期的原发感染可导致流产。妊娠将近足月时的感染可在分娩过程中传播给婴儿，导致高致死率及存活儿神经系统并发症的高发病率。妊娠足月原发感染或活动性复发感染是破膜前实施剖宫产的适应证。

其他病原体

沙眼衣原体和淋病奈瑟菌感染宫颈和子宫。它们很少传播至上生殖道，且无症状。

Herpes simplex virus (HSV)

Aetiology

Genital and anal herpes is usually caused by type II HSV, but type I HSV (usually responsible for oral cold sores) can also be a cause of genital infection. In the UK, genital HSV is the most common identifiable cause of genital ulceration.

Clinical features

A primary infection may present with prodromal discomfort, followed by the appearance of vesicles (Fig. 67), ulceration, inguinal lymphadenopathy together with malaise, fever and possibly urinary retention. In women the vesicles are usually situated on the vulva (Fig. 68), vagina and cervix. The lesions of a primary infection may take several weeks to heal and secondary infection is common. Recurrence of HSV infection is common, as the virus lies dormant in the posterior nerve root ganglia between recurrences. Recurrent infection is less florid. Diagnosis is made on clinical examination and confirmed by viral cultures from the ulcers.

Management

Aciclovir can be used to reduce symptoms and virus shedding times in a primary attack. It does not prevent recurrences except during continuous treatment.

Complications

Primary infection can give rise to systemic complications, including hepatitis, myelitis, encephalitis and meningitis. A primary infection in early pregnancy may cause abortion. Infection near term may be transmitted to the baby during delivery, leading to a high mortality rate and a high rate of neurological complications in the survivors. Primary infection or active recurrent disease at term are indications for delivery by caesarean section before rupture of the membranes.

Other pathogens

Chlamydia trachomatis and *Neisseria gonorrhoeae* infect the cervix and urethra. They are usually asymptomatic in the absence of spread to the upper genital tract.

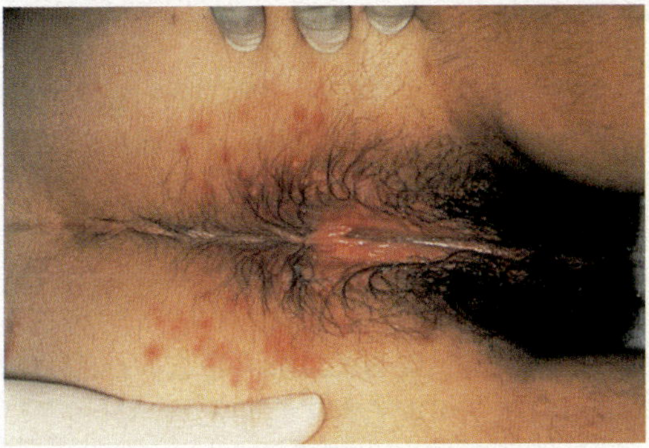

图 67　原发性生殖器疱疹感染
Primary genital herpes infection

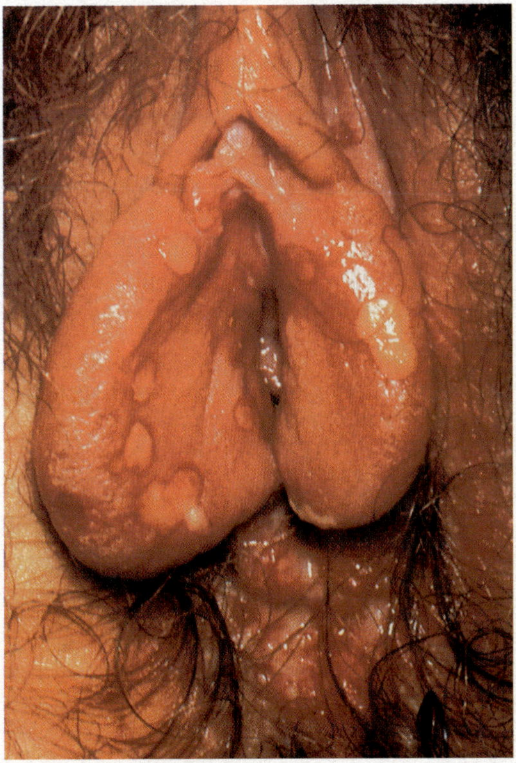

图 68　外阴疱疹感染
Vulval herpes infection

盆腔炎

定义	盆腔炎是由于下生殖道的病原微生物增殖，引起的子宫内膜、输卵管和 / 或临近组织的感染。
发病率	在英国每年大约有 100 000 的妇女患盆腔炎。大多数患者年龄不到 25 岁。
病因	年轻妇女中，绝大多数盆腔炎的病例与通过性传播的细菌感染有关，如沙眼衣原体和淋病奈瑟菌。这些细菌可能引起了病变，然后又被条件致病菌如链球菌和拟杆菌属所代替。
临床特征	临床表现为从隐性感染到明显症状和体征，如盆腔痛、性交痛、发热、阴道分泌物增多、热病、盆腔腹膜炎、宫颈刺激症状，还可能有盆腔肿物。右上腹痛可能由肝周炎引起（图 69）。15% 病例合并衣原体引起的盆腔炎。疑似病例中仅有65%可通过腹腔镜找到盆腔炎（图 70）的证据。
鉴别诊断	包括急性阑尾炎、子宫内膜炎、异位妊娠、卵巢囊肿急腹症和感染性肠病。
处理	抗生素联合应用能有效抵抗所有可能致病病原体，加上足量的止痛药是必要的。严重的病人需要住院治疗。如果保守治疗后病情没有改善或者恶化，就应当手术治疗。所有患盆腔炎的妇女及其性伴侣都应该去泌尿生殖诊所进行性传播疾病的检查及适当的治疗以避免再次感染。
并发症	15% ~ 20%的患者继发不孕症。患盆腔炎后，异位妊娠的风险可增高 7 ~ 10 倍。大约 20% 的妇女在盆腔炎后罹患慢性盆腔痛。

Pelvic inflammatory disease

Definition

An infection of the endometrium, fallopian tubes and/or contiguous structures caused by the ascent of microorganisms from the lower genital tract.

Incidence

Roughly 100 000 women in the UK develop PID each year. Most are less than 25 years of age.

Aetiology

The majority of cases of PID in young women are associated with sexually transmitted bacteria, e.g. *Chlamydia trachomatis and Neisseria gonorrhoeae*. These bacteria may initiate the process and then be replaced by opportunistic bacteria including streptococci and Bacteroides.

Clinical features

There is a spectrum of presentation from silent infection to florid symptoms and signs, e.g. pelvic pain, dyspareunia, fever, vaginal discharge, pyrexia, pelvic peritonism, cervical excitation and, possibly, a pelvic mass. Right upper quadrant pain may be due to perihepatitis (Fig. 69). It complicates up to 15% of cases of chlamydial PID. Laparoscopic evidence of PID (Fig. 70) is seen in only 65% of suspected cases.

Differential diagnosis

This includes acute appendicitis, endometriosis, ectopic pregnancy, ovarian cyst accident and inflammatory bowel conditions.

Management

A combination of antibiotics active against all likely causative organisms, along with adequate analgesia, are required. In severe cases, hospital admission may be necessary. Surgery is appropriate if the condition fails to improve or deteriorates with conservative management. All women with PID and their partners should be referred to a genitourinary medicine clinic, screened for sexually transmitted infections and treated appropriately to avoid reinfection.

Complications

Infertility follows in 15%~20% of cases. There is a seven- to 10-fold increased risk of an ectopic pregnancy, and chronic pelvic pain is suffered by roughly 20% of women after PID.

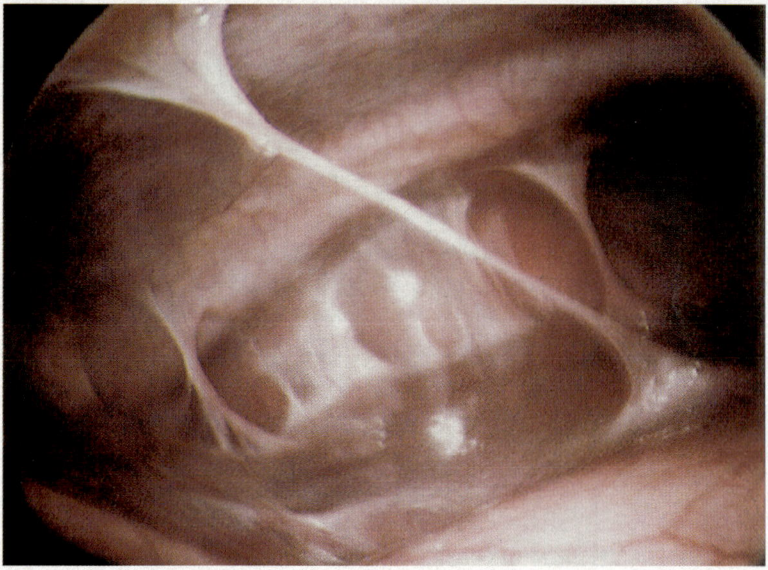

图 69　肝周粘连（Fitz-Hugh-Curtis 综合征）
Perihepatic adhesions (Fitz-Hugh-Curtis syndrome)

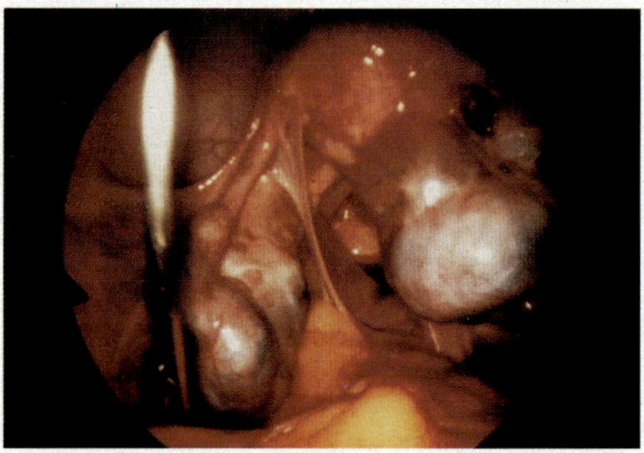

图 70　盆腔炎中双侧输卵管 - 卵巢脓肿
Bilateral tubo-ovarian abscesses in PID

HIV 感染

发病率和病因 人类免疫缺陷病毒（human immunodeficiency virus, HIV）广泛流行于南美、北美洲、亚撒哈拉非洲和西欧。年龄和性别分布差异很大。

传播方式

性传播 异性之间的性交是世界范围内最普遍的传播或获得HIV的方式。在欧洲和北美妇女在新发病例中比例增加。

非肠道途径 在1985年引进筛查和热疗前，通过血液、血制品和共用感染针头传播。

母婴传播 HIV抗体阳性的妇女生的孩子中11%～30%将会感染（如抗体持续存在18个月以上或在较早阶段有 HIV 的临床和免疫学表现）。在感染胎儿的传播中母体健康是重要因素。从母亲获得HIV的婴儿中大约有 25% 将会在一岁时发展为艾滋病。

临床特征 AIDS 被定义为由 HIV 引起的疾病，以一个或更多的“指示性”疾病为特征，这些疾病包括胃肠（图 71）和呼吸道念珠菌病、隐孢子虫病、肺孢子虫肺炎（图 72）和脑弓形虫病（图 73）。卡波西肉瘤（图74）在妇女中少见；其他疾病谱在男性和女性相似。

女性和 HIV

避孕方法的选择和怀孕的愿望是感染HIV的女性的重要问题。没有证据表明怀孕会加速患艾滋病的进程。复方口服避孕药可增加传播的风险，IUCD 可能会使 HIV 患者增加患盆腔感染性疾病的风险。

HIV infection

Incidence and aetiology

HIV (human immunodeficiency virus) is most prevalent in North and South America, sub-Saharan Africa and western Europe. The age and sex distribution varies widely.

Mode of transmission

Sexual Heterosexual intercourse is the most common mode of transmission/acquisition world wide. In Europe and North America, women are accounting for an increasing proportion of new cases.

Parenteral Spread is from blood and blood products, before screening and heat treatment were introduced in 1985, and from sharing infected needles.

Transmission from mother to fetus 11%~30% of children born to HIV-antibody-positive women will be infected (i.e. have antibodies persisting for more than 18 months or develop clinical and or immunological manifestations of HIV at an earlier stage). Maternal health is an important factor in transmission of infection to the fetus. Of those infants who acquire HIV from their mothers, about 25% will develop AIDS in the first year of life.

Clinical features

AIDS is defined as an illness caused by HIV and characterized by one or more 'indicator' diseases, which include candidiasis of the gastrointestinal (Fig. 71) and respiratory tract, cryptosporidiosis, *Pneumocystis carinii* pneumonia (Fig. 72) and toxoplasmosis of the brain (Fig. 73). Kaposi's sarcoma (Fig. 74) is rare in women; otherwise the spectrum of disease seen in men and women is similar.

Women and HIV

Important issues for women with HIV concern choice of contraception and wishes regarding pregnancy. There is no evidence that pregnancy accelerates the progress to AIDS. It has been suggested that the combined oral contraceptive pill may increase the risk of transmission and that an IUCD may put women with HIV at increased risk of pelvic inflammatory disease.

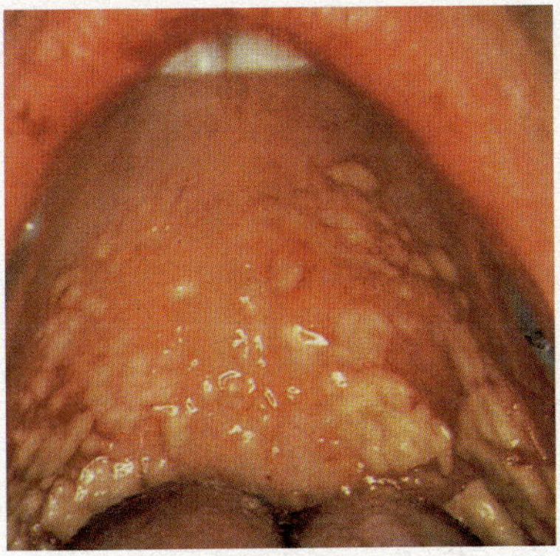

图 71　口腔念珠菌病
Oral candidiasis

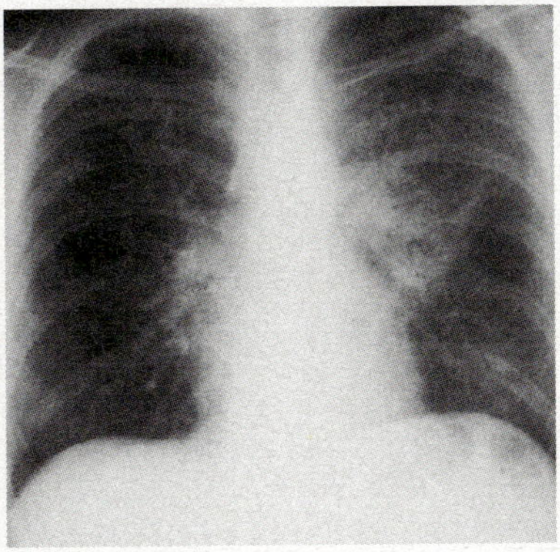

图 72　卡他肺孢子虫肺炎
Pneumocystis carinii pneumonia

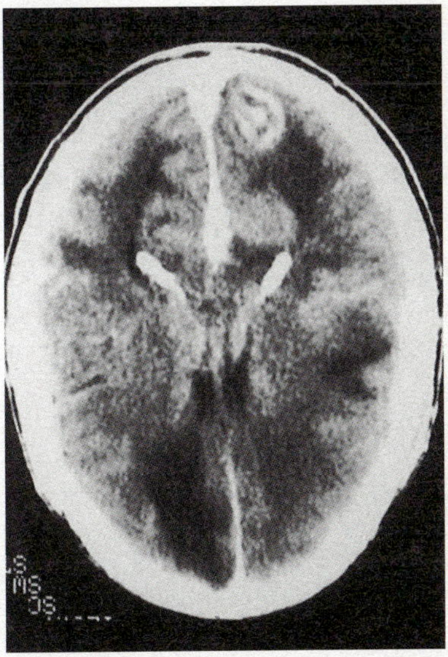

图 73　脑弓形虫病
Cerebral toxoplasmosis

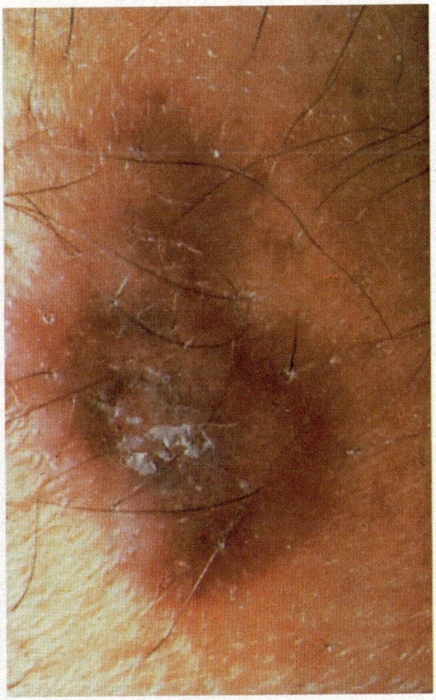

图 74　卡波西肉瘤
Kaposi's sarcoma

9 子宫内膜异位症

定义

子宫内膜异位症是一种良性疾病，特征是子宫内膜组织在子宫腔以外的部位存在和增殖。

发病率

10%以上绝经前的高加索妇女和30%表现为不孕的女性。口服避孕药的应用可减少子宫内膜异位症的发生。

病因

关于子宫内膜异位症的发病机理有很多理论，但没有一种可以解释所有的病例。因此，形成了以下多种理论联合的局面：

- *经血逆流*：月经期子宫内膜组织沿着输卵管种植在腹腔
- *淋巴和血行播散*：子宫内膜组织在远处部位导致栓塞
- *体腔上皮化生*：腹腔内月经血的反复炎性损害可以导致腹膜组织的分化和有活力的内膜组织的生长

病理

是由炎症、纤维化和粘连形成构成的非感染性过程。整个外观呈黑色斑点（粉末烧灼状）（图 75），多出现在卵巢表面、宫骶韧带（图76）和直肠子宫陷凹。粘连形成和正常解剖结构的扭转可能是病情严重的特征（图 77）。如果病变累及卵巢，可形成“巧克力囊肿”。子宫内膜异位症的不常见部位包括脐、剖腹手术瘢痕、外阴切开术瘢痕、宫颈、直肠、膀胱、肺、大腿和外阴。

临床表现

包括疼痛，可能为周期性疼痛、性交困难、背痛和继发性痛经。膀胱或直肠受累导致的血尿或直肠出血少见。子宫内膜异位症也可无症状。

Endometriosis 9

Definition

Endometriosis is a benign process characterized by the presence and proliferation of endometrial tissue in sites outside the uterine cavity.

Incidence

It is seen in up to 10% of premenopausal Caucasian women and 30% of women presenting with infertility. The use of the oral contraceptive pill reduces the incidence of endometriosis.

Aetiology

A number of theories regarding the pathogenesis of endometriosis exist, but no single theory will explain all cases. The condition may therefore result from a combination of the following:

- *Retrograde menstruation*: the passage of endometrial tissue along the fallopian tubes during menstruation with implantation in the peritoneal cavity
- *Lymphatic or vascular spread*: endometrial tissue embolizing to distant sites
- *Metaplasia of coelomic epithelium*: the repeated inflammatory insult from menstrual blood in the peritoneal cavity may lead to redifferentiation of the peritoneal tissue and the development of viable endometrial tissue

Pathology

A non-infectious process of inflammation, fibrosis and adhesion formation. The gross appearance is of black spots ('powder burns') (Fig. 75), commonly on the ovaries, uterosacral ligaments (Fig. 76) and pouch of Douglas. Adhesion formation and distortion of normal anatomy may be a feature in severe disease (Fig. 77). If the ovaries are involved, 'chocolate cysts' may form. Unusual sites for endometriosis include the umbilicus, laparotomy scars, episiotomy scars, cervix, bowel, bladder, lung, thigh and vulva.

Clinical features

These include pain, which may be cyclical, dyspareunia, backache and secondary dysmenorrhoea. Rarely there may be haematuria or rectal bleeding if the bladder or bowel are involved. Endometriosis may also be symptomless.

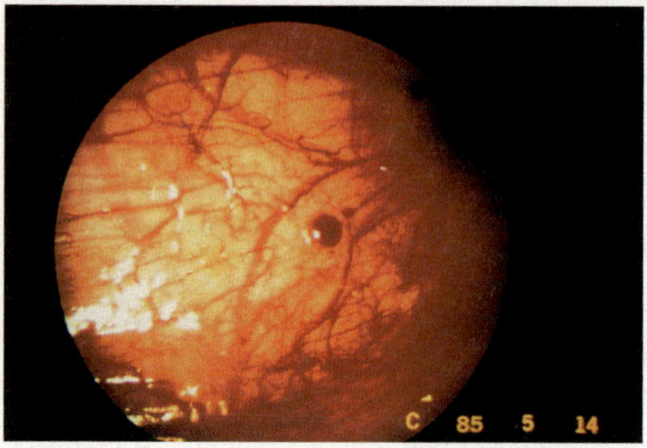

图 75　子宫内膜异位灶
Endometriotic deposit

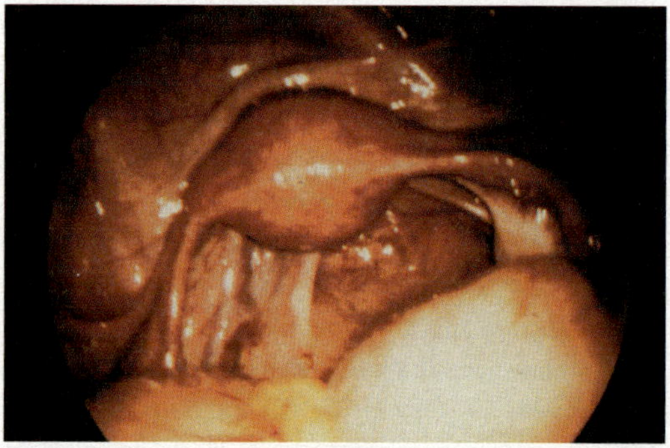

图 76　腹腔镜显示在左侧的极小的子宫内膜异位症
Laparoscopy showing minimal endometriosis on left

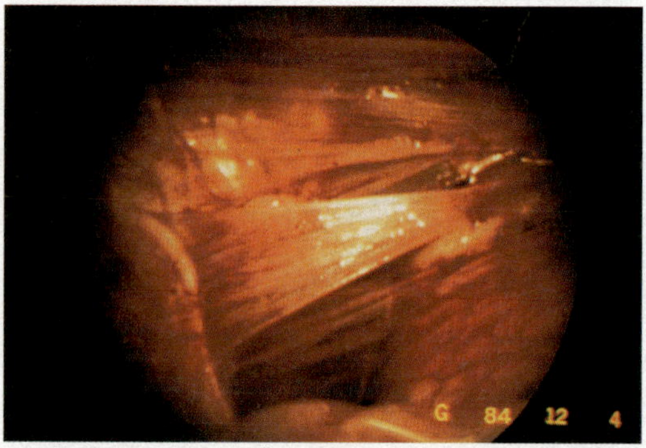

图 77　继发于子宫内膜异位症的粘连
Adhesions secondary to endometriosis

检查

全面的临床检查是必要的，可以发现局部的子宫内膜沉积，如宫颈子宫内膜异位症（图 78）。

辅助检查

确诊靠腹腔镜（图79）或剖腹术。如果以血尿或直肠出血为特征，则有必要行膀胱镜、乙状结肠镜检查和钡剂灌肠。

处理

有症状的病例可以用药物或手术治疗。

药物治疗

基于妊娠可使异位子宫内膜改善，可连续口服避孕药9个月撤退性出血且不停药，以模拟妊娠。孕激素如醋酸甲羟孕酮，也可以抑制排卵和缓解症状。达那唑（一种睾酮衍生物）可以产生高雄激素、低雌激素环境而不支持子宫内膜的生长。孕三烯酮作用与达那唑相同，优点是每周服药两次而不用每天服两次药。GnRH类似物可以鼻内或皮下给药，在下丘脑水平抑制排卵。

在子宫内膜异位症的治疗中许多药物治疗是有效的，但不幸的是病情可能复发。所有药物都会产生副作用：口服避孕药的突破性出血；孕激素的胃胀气和经前期样综合征；达那唑的促男性化副作用；以及GnRH类似物引起的低雌激素反应如潮热和骨质疏松（这些症状可以应用“反向添加”治疗来消除）。药物治疗必须要个体化用药。

手术治疗

手术方法可通过腹腔镜（电透热疗法或激光切除和分离粘连）或剖腹术修补盆腔解剖或切除子宫和卵巢。

Examination

A thorough clinical examination is essential and may reveal localized endometrial deposits, e.g. cervical endometriosis (Fig. 78).

Investigations

The definitive diagnosis is made by laparoscopy (Fig. 79) or laparotomy. If haematuria or rectal bleeding are features, cystoscopy, sigmoidoscopy and barium enema would be necessary.

Management

Symptomatic disease can be treated medically or surgically.

Medical treatment

Medicial treatment is based on the observation that endometriosis improves in pregnancy. The use of the oral contraceptive pill, without breaks for withdrawal bleeds, for up to 9 months mimics pregnancy and is associated with symptomatic improvement. Progestogens, e.g. medroxyprogesterone acetate, also suppress ovulation and give relief from symptoms. Danazol (a testosterone derivative) creates a high-androgen, low-oestrogen environment that does not support the growth of endometrium. Gestrinone acts similarly to danazol and has the advantage of being taken twice weekly as opposed to twice daily. GnRH analogues given intranasally or subcutaneously suppress ovulation at the hypothalamus.

Many medical treatments are effective in the treatment of endometriosis but unfortunately the condition can relapse. Side effects arise with all medications: breakthrough bleeding on the oral contraceptive pill; bloating and PMS-like symptoms with progestogen; androgenic side effects with danazol; and hypooestrogenic effects such as hot flushes and bone loss with GnRH analogues. (These can be counteracted with 'add-back' therapy.) Medical treatment must be tailored to the individual patient.

Surgical treatment

Surgical approaches can be through the laparoscope (diathermy or laser ablation and division of adhesions) or by laparotomy to restore pelvic anatomy or remove the uterus and ovaries.

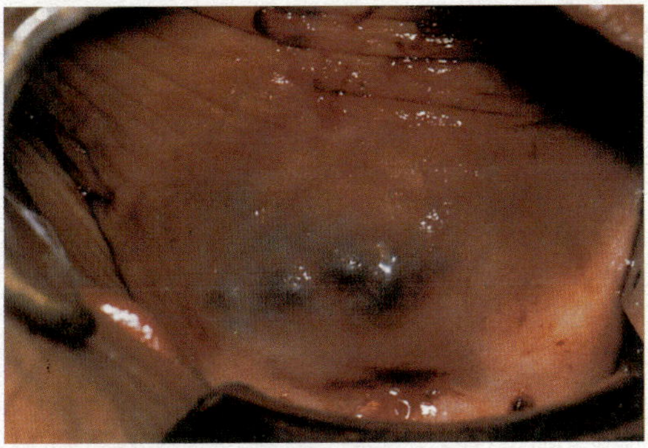

图 78　宫颈子宫内膜异位症
Cervical endometriosis

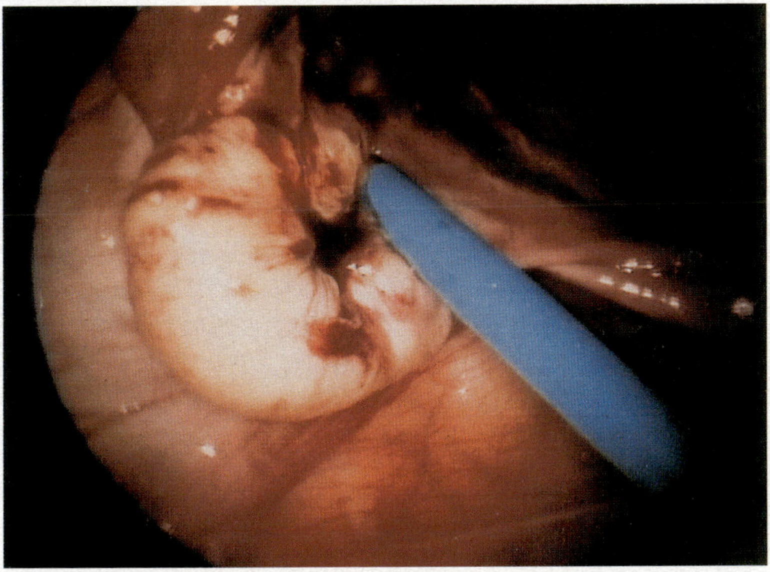

图 79　腹腔镜下分离子宫内膜异位症粘连
Laparoscopic division of endometriotic adhesion

10 不孕症

定义

规律的无防护性生活超过 12 个月而未能受孕诊断为不孕症。1/6 的夫妇会受到影响。

病因

不孕症的三个主要原因：精液质量差、输卵管异常和排卵紊乱。其他罕见的原因包括宫颈黏液异常和抗精子抗体、阳痿和逆射精。有些不能解释的不孕症占很大比例（10% ~ 20%），包括心理因素。

临床特征

通过夫妻双方详尽的病史可得知病因。对于女性，排卵的证据可以通过月经周期的规律和相关的症状，如疼痛、宫颈黏液的改变和原发性痛经而获得。输卵管异常通常继发于炎症（图80，81）或盆腔手术（如卵巢囊肿切除术）的瘢痕和粘连。除此之外，子宫内膜异位症也可引起盆腔瘢痕。如果输卵管远端阻塞，可形成输卵管积水（图 82）。如果有使用宫内节育器、盆腔炎、盆腔手术或有盆腔痛的病史，应疑有输卵管损伤。

检查可显示内分泌紊乱（如多囊卵巢综合征或过早绝经的组织萎缩）和盆腔病理学特征（如子宫内膜异位征瘢痕、卵巢囊肿或纤维瘤）。

对于男性，病史可以提示既往的手术史或感染史。应激和近期所患疾病可能与短暂的精液质量下降有关。

检查应包括睾丸，以寻找静脉曲张或输精管缺如。由于纤维化而导致的睾丸体积减小和硬度增加可有生精障碍。附睾肿胀可提示输精管阻塞。

罕见的无精子症可能由于促性腺激素分泌不足性性腺机能减退引起，它表现为缺少第二性征。

Definition

Failure to conceive after 12 months of regular unprotected intercourse. 1:6 couples affected.

Aetiology

Three main causes of infertility: poor semen quality, tubal disorders and ovulatory disorders. Other rarer causes include mucus 'hostility' and sperm antibodies, impotence and retrograde ejaculation. This leaves a significant (10%~20%) proportion with unexplained infertility, which includes psychological factors.

Clinical features

Significant clues to the aetiology can be achieved by a thorough history from both partners. In the female, evidence of ovulation can be gained from regularity of menstrual cycle and associated symptoms, e.g. mittleschmerz pain, cervical mucus changes and primary dysmenorrhoea.
Tubal disorders are usually the result of scarring and adhesions secondary to infection (Figs 80, 81) or pelvic surgery, e.g. ovarian cystectomy. In addition, endometriosis may cause pelvic scarring. If the distal portion of the tube is blocked, a hydrosalpinx may develop (Fig. 82). Tubal damage should be suspected if there is a history of IUCD use, PID, pelvic surgery or pelvic pain.
Examination may also reveal endocrinological disorders, e.g. PCOS, or the tissue atrophy of premature menopause, and physical signs of pelvic pathology, e.g. endometriotic scarring, ovarian cysts or fibroids.
In the male, history may reveal previous operations or infections. Stress and recent intercurrent illnesses may be associated with transitory reduced semen quality.
Examination should include testicles, looking for varicosities or the absence of the vas deferens. Reduced testicular size and increased firmness due to fibrosis may indicate spermatogenic failure. A swollen epididymis may indicate a blockage of the vas.
Rarely, azoospermia may be due to hypogonadotrophic hypogonadism, indicated by lack of secondary sexual development.

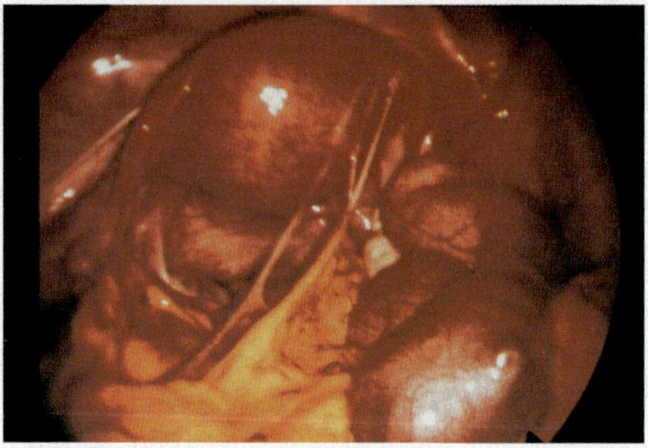

图 80　盆腔炎后的盆腔粘连
Pelvic adhesions after PID

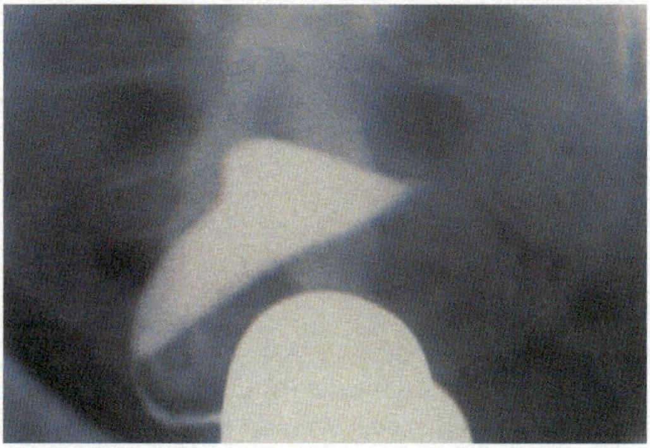

图 81　宫角阻塞
Cornual blockage

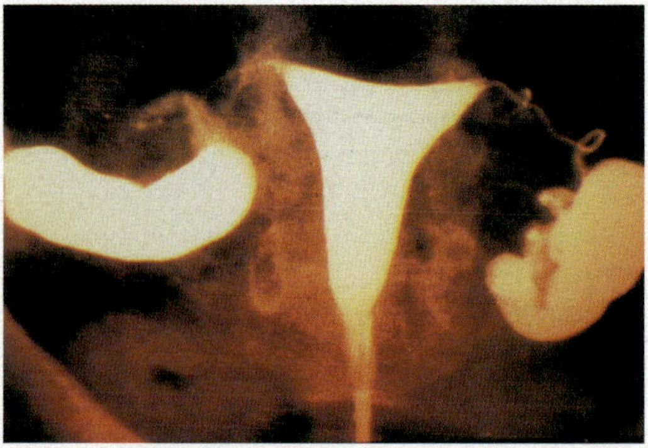

图 82　双侧输卵管积水
Bilateral hydrosalpinges

鉴别诊断

确定不孕症的特定原因需要恰当的病史和体检及如下所述的适当的检查。

检查

男性

对于男性，两次精液分析是基本检查。正常的精液分析，WHO 标准是精子密度⩾ 2000 万 / 毫升，其中有⩾ 50% 为向前运动的精子并且⩾ 50% 精子为正常形态。此标准与正常的受孕率有关。如果精液分析值降低，则可提示血清 LH、FSH 和睾酮含量变化。高促性腺激素表明睾丸功能障碍。精液分析值正常而睾酮水平减低提示促性腺激素分泌不足性性腺功能减退。在非梗阻性和一些梗阻性的无精子症中可以用睾丸活检来评估精子产生和精子储备量。

女性

对于女性，应进行简单的排卵检测，如测量黄体中期血清孕酮含量、画不超过两个月经周期的基础体温图（图 83）。更加复杂的检查包括超声下监测卵泡（图 84）和连续的 LH 检测来检查排卵前的 LH 脉冲，以及黄体期腹腔镜检查证实黄体的存在。

腹腔镜和染料注入法（图85）是最佳的检查输卵管未闭或破坏的方法，另外，此方法还具有盆腔显像的优点，如显示卵巢（黄体存在）、腹膜以除外子宫内膜异位灶，以及子宫来评价其解剖异常。我们用子宫输卵管造影术来评定输卵管是否通畅，也可显示子宫内病变如粘连、纤维化或诸如双角子宫（图 86）的解剖学异常。其他的检查包括性交后实验可评估精子在宫颈黏液中的活动能力、夫妻双方和丈夫精液中的抗精子抗体。

Differential diagnosis

Defining the specific causes of infertility requires a proper history and examination and appropriate investigations as outlined below.

Investigations

Male

For the male, a semen analysis on two occasions is the basic investigation. The WHO criteria for a normal semen analysis is a sperm density of $\geqslant$ 20 million sperm per mL with $\geqslant$ 50% sperm with forward progression and $\geqslant$ 50% normal morphology. The criteria are associated with a normal rate of conception. If the values are reduced, serum LH, FSH and testosterone are indicated. High gonadotrophins are indicative of testicular failure. Normal levels with reduced testosterone may indicate hypogonadotrophic hypogonadism. In cases of non-obstructive and some cases of obstructive azoospermia there may be an indication for testicular biopsy to assess spermatogenesis and storage of any sperm found for future use.

Female

In the female, simple tests for ovulation should be undertaken, i.e. mid-luteal phase serum progesterone, basal body temperature charts (Fig. 83) for no more than two cycles. More sophisticated investigations include follicle monitoring with ultrasound (Fig. 84), serial LH measurements to detect the pre-ovulatory LH surge, and laparoscopy in the luteal phase to confirm the presence of a corpus luteum.

Laparoscopy and dye instillation (Fig. 85) provide the optimum test of tubal patency or damage with the additional benefit of visualization of the pelvis, i.e. ovaries (for the presence of corpus luteum), peritoneum to exclude endometriotic deposits, and the uterus to assess anatomical abnormality. Hysterosalpingography is used to assess tubal patency and also to reveal intrauterine problems, e.g. adhesions, fibroids or anatomical abnormalities such as bicornuate uterus (Fig. 86). Other investigations include a postcoital test, which assesses the capacity of sperm to remain motile in the cervical mucus, and tests for antisperm antibodies in both partners and in the husband's seminal plasma.

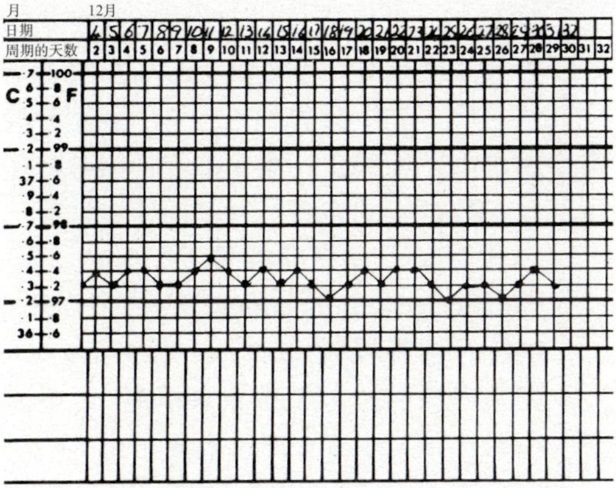

图 83　体温图缺少黄体期体温上升值，显示无排卵图形
Temperature chart showing an anovulatory pattern with absence of luteal phase rise

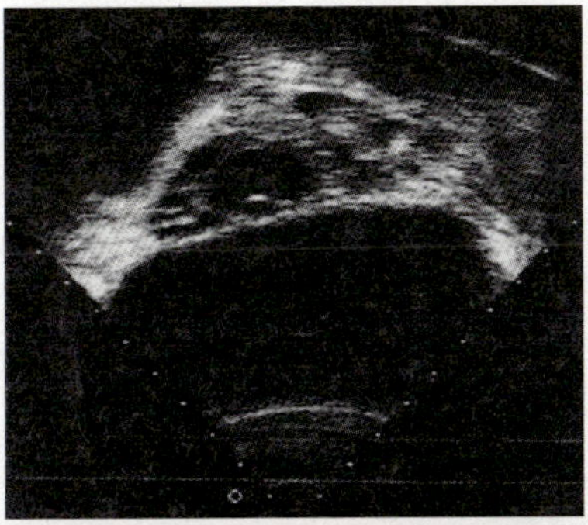

图 84　超声下的优势卵泡图像
Ultrasound image of a dominant follicle

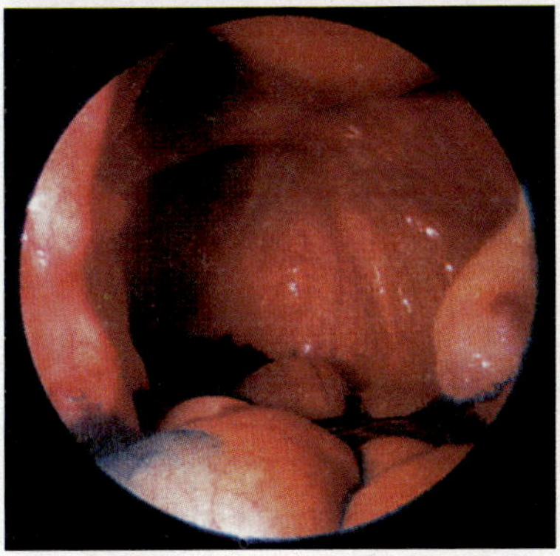

图 85　盆腔内通过蓝染显示输卵管通畅
Tubal patency as shown by presence of blue dye in the pelvis

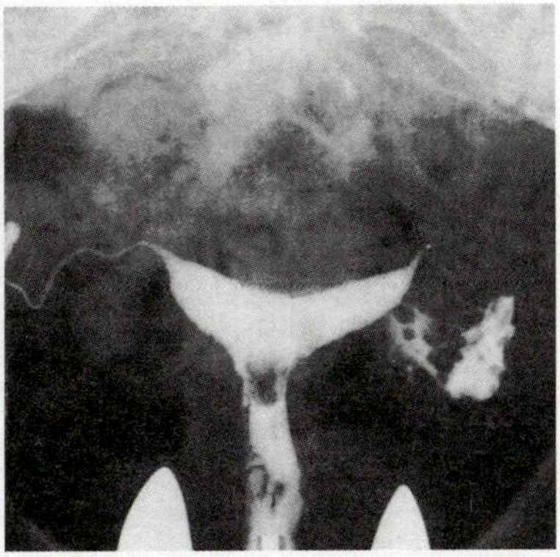

图 86　双角子宫的子宫输卵管造影
Hysterosalpingogram of bicornuate uterus

治疗

男性

过去，精液质量低下者很少有机会改善，除非是短暂的病症如应激或病毒感染。精索静脉曲张修补术的价值还不确定。激素治疗还未被证实有效。对于精子数量少的患者，目前治疗方法有：准备小剂量的优质精子在排卵期置于子宫内（子宫内受精，intrauterine insemination，IUI）或从患者体内取卵母细胞行体外授精（in vitro fertilization，IVF）。精子卵浆内注射技术（intracytoplasmic sperm injection，ICSI）显著改善了严重的男子不育症的治疗效果。ICSI仅需少量的精子，可用于梗阻性和非梗阻性无精子症的治疗。有抗精子抗体的男性患者可使用类固醇激素而被成功治疗。但供者的精液仍然是许多男性不育症的唯一选择。

女性

排卵障碍对激素（如克罗米酚或人绝经期促性腺激素）治疗反应好。使用人绝经期促性腺激素要求严密监测以避免过度刺激或多胎妊娠。在选择性病例中可通过手术（图87）治疗输卵管损伤，但其成功率很少超过 30%。

IVF技术的成功率为20% ~ 25%。它包括刺激卵巢产生大量的卵泡，从这些卵泡中吸取卵母细胞与丈夫的精子行体外授精，受精后48~72小时再将受精卵移植至宫腔。

对于宫颈黏液阻碍受精或未发现原因的不孕症，如无法解释的不孕症，IVF和输卵管内配子移植术（gamete intrafallopian transfer，GIFT。图88）等助孕技术是可行的。成功率为 25% ~ 30%。

并发症

与应用药物和介入手术不同，其主要并发症是不能怀孕造成的心理创伤。在许多夫妇中发病率较高，他们需要心理咨询和支持使他们能够适应无子女的情况。

Management

Male

Poor semen quality previously had little opportunity for improvement unless it was a transitory problem, e.g. stress or viral infection. The value of varicocele repair is unresolved. Hormonal treatments are unproven. With low counts, options that are now available include the preparation of a small volume of the best sperm to place within the uterus at ovulation (intrauterine insemination; IUI) or in vitro fertilization (IVF) with oocytes collected from the patient. Intracytoplasmic sperm injection or ICSI has dramatically altered the treatment of severe male factor infertility. ICSI only requires low sperm numbers and can be used in the treatment of both obstructive and non-obstructive azoospermia. Antisperm antibodies have been successfully treated with steroids in the male. Donor semen remains the only option for many infertile men.

Female

Ovulatory disorders respond well to hormonal therapy, i.e. clomiphene or human menopausal gonadotrophins. The latter requires close monitoring to avoid hyperstimulation or high-order multiple pregnancy. Tubal damage can be dealt with by surgery (Fig. 87) in selected cases, but the results rarely exceed 30%.

Bypassing the tube with IVF is successful in 20%~25% of cycles. This involves ovarian stimulation to produce multiple follicles, the aspiration of the oocytes from these follicles, the in vitro fertilization with partner's semen and transfer to the uterus 48~72h after fertilization.

Assisted conception techniques including IVF and gamete intrafallopian transfer (GIFT: Fig. 88) are also applicable where mucus hostility is a possible cause or where no cause is found, e.g. unexplained infertility. Success rates in these groups are 25%~30%.

Complications

The major complication of infertility other than those associated with drugs and surgical intervention is the psychological trauma of being unable to conceive. Significant morbidity is present in many couples, who require counselling and support to enable them to come to terms with childlessness.

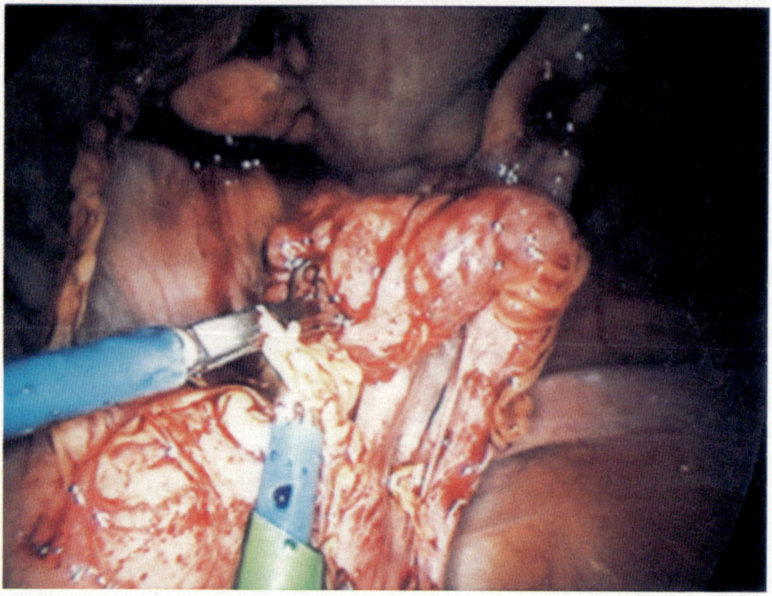

图 87　腹腔镜下游离盆腔粘连
Laparoscopic freeing of pelvic adhesions

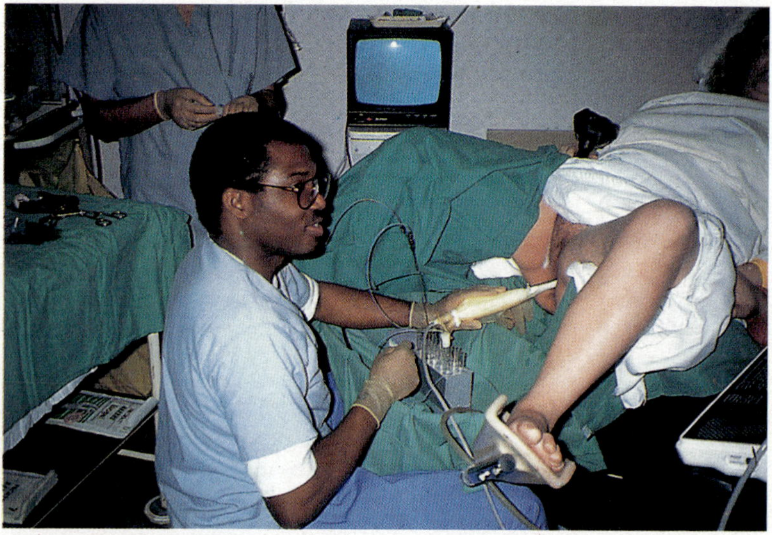

图 88　吸取卵母细胞行 IVF
Oocytes being aspirated for IVF

多囊卵巢综合征 11

定义

多囊卵巢综合征（polycystic ovarian syndrome，PCOS）是一种包括月经稀发、多毛（图89，90）、肥胖和不孕的综合征；它与垂体后叶促性腺激素分泌和卵巢类固醇产生紊乱有关。它是一个疾病谱，月经周期正常的妇女可能也有多囊卵巢，还可无以上症状。

发病率

根据不同的使用标准（临床或超声），妇女发病率为5% ~ 30%。在闭经的妇女中，30% ~ 40%可能有PCOS。在多毛的女性中发病率上升到50% ~ 70%。

病因

PCOS的病因还未确定。有两种主要的假说：

- 卵巢酶异常导致激素产生异常
- 垂体后叶素引起的反馈机制紊乱导致促性腺激素分泌异常和继发性卵巢功能障碍

少数PCOS病例表现为家族性，病因为卵巢酶异常。其净结果是LH分泌增加、不排卵和卵巢雄激素生成增加。

病理

典型的多囊卵巢体积增加是由于：

- 间质组织增加
- 多个卵巢囊泡，直径在2 ~ 4mm，分布在卵巢周围（珍珠结节，图91）

临床表现

通常从儿童期就表现为肥胖，而多毛通常出现在青春期，发生在面部、胸部和腹部。月经稀发表现在青春期，经常伴随偶发的继发性闭经。不孕症通常是原发性的。

11 Polycystic ovarian syndrome

Definition

Polycystic ovarian syndrome (PCOS) is a syndrome that consists of oligomenorrhoea, hirsutism (Figs 89, 90), obesity and infertility; it is associated with disordered pituitary gonadotrophin secretion and ovarian steroid production. It is a spectrum of disease as normally cycling women may have polycystic ovaries and yet none of the features above.

Incidence

Depending on the criteria used (clinical or ultrasound), the incidence varies from 5%~30% of the female population. Amongst amenorrhoeic women, 30%~40% probably have PCOS. Amongst hirsute women that incidence rises to 50%~70%.

Aetiology

The cause of PCOS is uncertain. There are two main hypotheses:

- ovarian enzyme abnormality resulting in abnormal steroid production
- disordered feedback mechanisms acting on the pituitary, resulting in abnormal gonadotrophin secretion with secondary ovarian dysfunction

A small proportion of PCOS cases have been shown to be familial and due to ovarian enzyme abnormalities. The net result is an increased LH secretion, anovulation and increased ovarian androgen production.

Pathology

The classic polycystic ovary is increased in size due to:

- increased stromal tissue
- multiple ovarian cysts, 2~4 mm in diameter, distributed around the periphery of the ovary (pearl nodi; Fig. 91)

Clinical features

Obesity is usually present from childhood, while hirsutism usually appears at puberty, affecting the face, chest and abdomen. Oligomenorrhoea is present from puberty, often with episodes of secondary amenorrhoea. Infertility is usually primary.

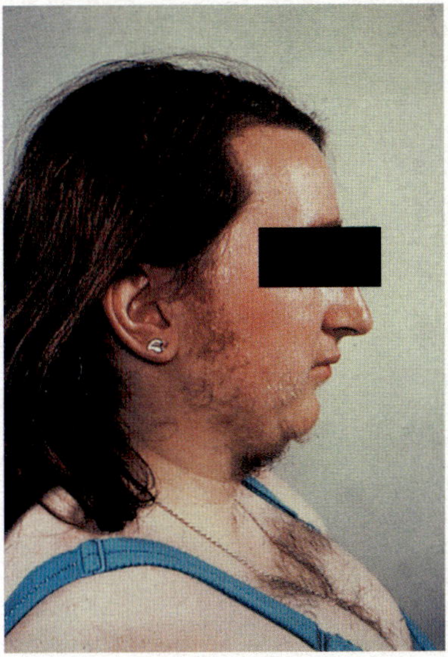

图 89 治疗前的多毛
Hirsutism before treatment

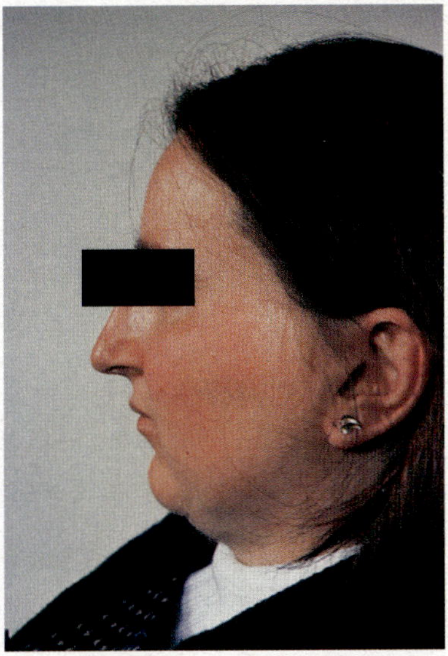

图 90 图89同一患者在激素治疗后
Same patient as in Figure 89 after hormone treatment

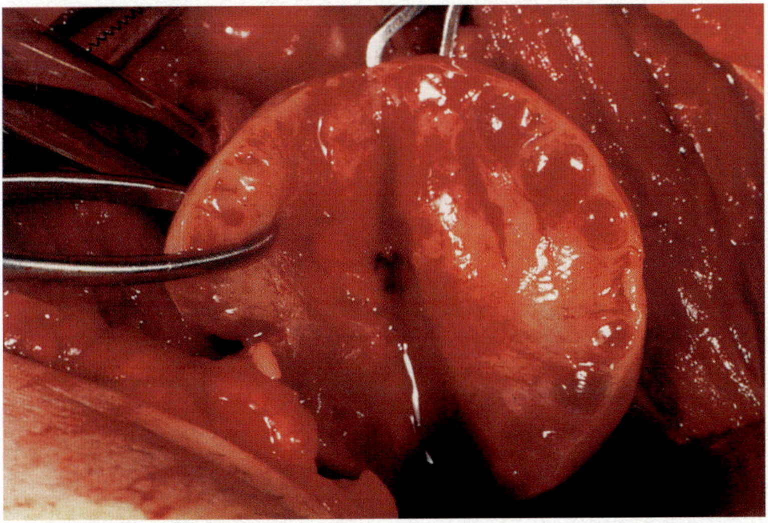

图 91 多囊卵巢的切面
Cut surface of polycystic ovary

鉴别诊断

肾上腺雄激素产生增加可能也意味着:

- 库欣综合征
- 肾上腺增生
- 肾上腺肿瘤

多毛可能也是家族性的，或由于药物引起，而其他的继发性闭经的原因包括高泌乳素血症。不孕症的其他原因可见相关内容。

检查

生化检查 血清LH、FSH、泌乳素、睾酮（硫酸脱氢表雄酮、雄烯二酮）。

超声 卵巢和盆腔（图92）（腹腔镜）。

处理

多毛 治疗包括:

- 美容治疗（膏剂、上蜡和电解除毛）
- 口服有低雄激素作用的孕激素的避孕药
- 抗雄激素（环丙孕酮醋酸盐）和安体舒通

肥胖 通过饮食控制 ± 二甲双胍

月经稀发/闭经 治疗包括:

- 口服避孕药以产生规律的撤退性出血
- 克罗米酚（50%患者将产生规律月经周期并将诱发排卵）

不孕症 克罗米酚诱导排卵在PCOS妇女中成功率为70%～80%，妊娠率与规律排卵的妇女相同。如果没有成功排卵，通过使用HMG、LHRH类似物（不论能否使垂体激素下调）通常都是有效的。后者将可导致严重的卵巢过度刺激（图93）。

并发症 这组肥胖和不排卵妇女往后很可能发展为子宫内膜异常增生和腺癌。孕激素或口服避孕药诱导的子宫内膜规律脱落似乎是合理的，尽管还没有被证实其预防作用。

Differential diagnosis

Increased adrenal androgen production could also mean:

- Cushing syndrome
- adrenal hyperplasia
- adrenal carcinoma

Hirsutism could also be familial, or due to drugs, while other causes of secondary amenorrhoea include hyperprolactinaemia. Other causes of infertility can be found on page 64.

Investigation

Biochemical Serum LH, FSH, prolactin, testosterone (DHEAS, androstenedione).

Ultrasound Ovaries and pelvis (Fig. 92) (laparoscopy).

Management

Hirsutism Management includes:

- cosmetic treatments (cream, waxing and electrolysis)
- oral contraceptive pill with low androgenic progestogen
- anti-androgens (cyproterone acetate) and spironolactone

Obesity is treated with diet ± metformin.

Oligoamenorrhoea/amenorrhoea Treatment includes:

- oral contraceptive pill to produce regular withdrawal bleeds
- clomiphene (will produce regular cycles in 50% but will also induce ovulation)

Infertility Induction of ovulation with clomiphene is successful in 70%~80% of women with PCOS, with pregnancy rates equivalent to regularly ovulating women. If not successful, HMG, with or without pituitary downregulation using LHRH analogues, is usually effective. This latter regime can result in severe ovarian hyperstimulation (Fig. 93).

Complications

This group of obese, anovulatory women are more likely to develop endometrial hyperplasia and adenocarcinoma in later life. Regular shedding of the endometrium induced by progestogens or the oral contraceptive pill seems a logical, though unproven, prophylaxis.

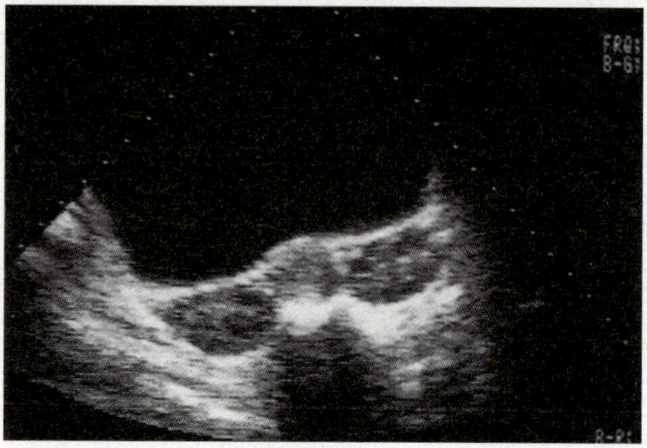

图 92　超声显示多囊卵巢
Ultrasound showing polycystic ovaries

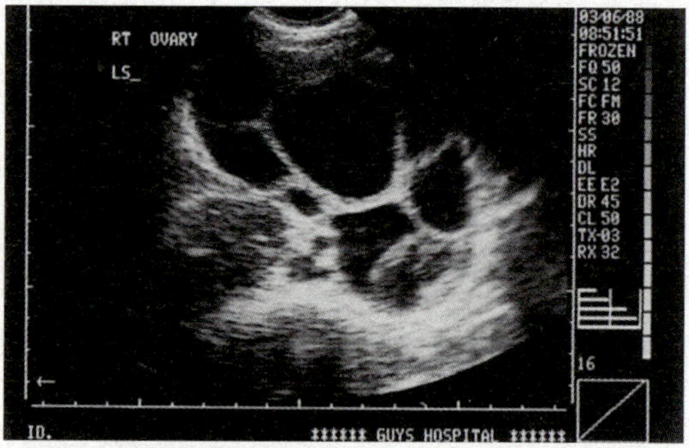

图 93　超声所见多囊卵巢的过度刺激
Hyperstimulation in a polycystic ovary as seen by ultrasound

外阴和阴道良、恶性疾病

外阴瘙痒

病因

任何年龄的患者都可能产生外阴瘙痒，原因很多。老年妇女最常见的原因是感染、雌激素缺乏和外阴皮肤病。

病理

最常见的感染原是假丝酵母菌。非感染性病因包括苔藓性硬化（图94）、Paget病和外阴上皮内瘤样病变（vulval intraepithelial neoplasia，VIN）。外阴Paget病常见于老年妇女（图95）。VIN是浸润癌的先兆。

临床特征

可出现外阴刺激和瘙痒。检查时可能出现表皮脱落、变色（图 94）以及外阴皮肤变厚或变薄。

巴氏腺体

这两个腺体结构位于阴道口后方深部。它们可能被感染，表现为大而软的脓肿。治疗方法是造口术。腺体也可能出现囊肿（图 96）。

尿道肉阜

尿道外口凸出（图97）并肿胀。可能会出血或组织很脆。尿道肉阜常合并感染。如果手术治疗，切除的组织应该送组织学检查以排除尿道癌。

尖锐湿疣

性病疣状物常见于外阴（图66）或阴道内。这些疣可以通过局部用药、局部去除或手术治疗。

12 Benign and malignant conditions of the vulva and vagina

Pruritus vulvae

Aetiology

Vulval irritation can occur at any age, and the causes are numerous. The most common are infection, oestrogen deficiency and vulval dermatoses in the older woman.

Pathology

The most common infective agent is Candida. Non-infectious causes include lichen sclerosus (Fig. 94), Paget's disease and vulval intraepithelial neoplasia (VIN). Paget's disease of the vulva usually presents in the elderly (Fig. 95). VIN is a precursor of invasive carcinoma.

Clinical features

Irritation and itchiness of the vulva are present. On examination there may be evidence of excoriation, discoloration (Fig. 94), thickening or thinning of the vulval skin.

Bartholin's glands

These are paired structures that lie deep to the posterior introitus. They can become infected and present as a large, tender, swollen abscess. Marsupialization is the treatment of choice. Cyst formation can also occur (Fig. 96).

Urethral caruncle

The external urethral meatus protrudes (Fig. 97) and swells. It may bleed, and may be very tender. Urethral caruncles are often associated with infection. If surgery is performed, the excised piece of tissue should be sent for histological confirmation to exclude urethral carcinoma.

Condylomata acuminata

Venereal warts are common on the vulva (Fig. 66) or in the vagina. They can be treated by topical applications, local destructive methods or surgery.

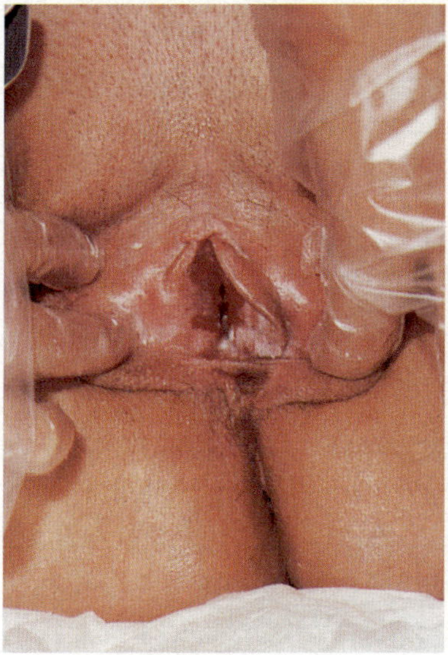

图 94　苔藓性硬化
Lichen sclerosus

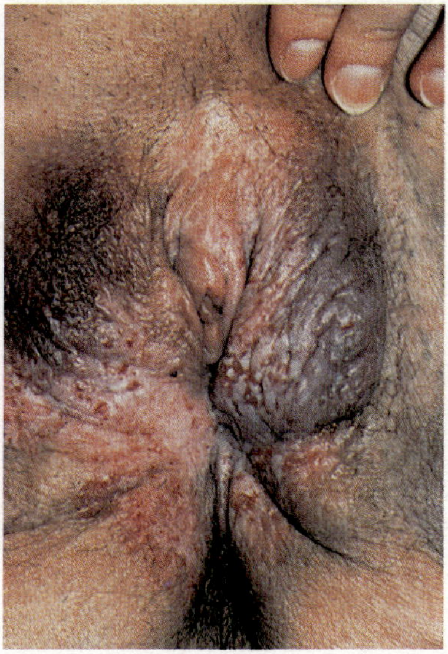

图 95　外阴 Paget 病
Paget's disease of the vulva

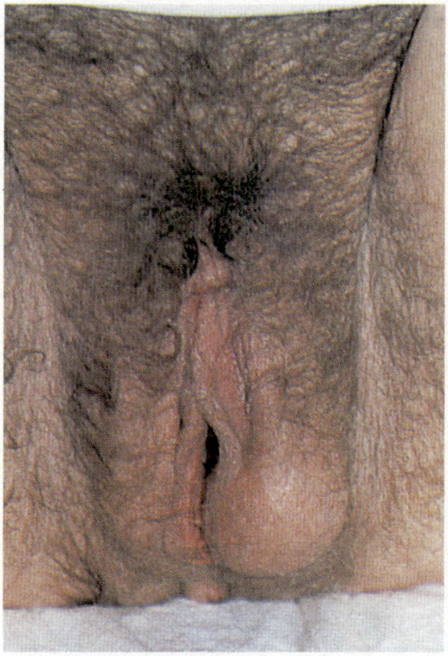

图 96　巴氏腺囊肿
Bartholin's cyst

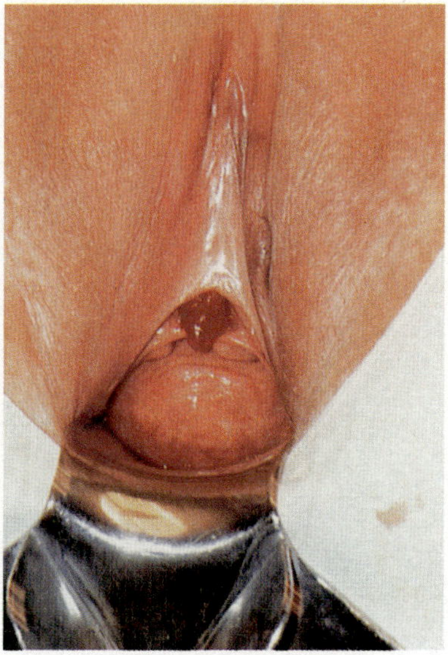

图 97　尿道肉阜合并膀胱膨出
Urethral caruncle with cystocele

外阴癌

病因及发病率 外阴癌不常见，通常限于老年妇女并伴有深部的外阴状况异常，如硬化萎缩性苔藓。然而，年轻妇女携带高危型 HPV 病毒和吸烟者患病率有所增加。

病理 外阴癌（图98）通常生长缓慢，大多为鳞状细胞肿瘤。大多淋巴回流直接进入腹股沟浅、深淋巴结，然后进入髂淋巴。基底细胞癌和黑色素瘤少见。

临床特征 通常表现为肿块或溃疡，并有瘙痒史。

处理 所有可疑的病灶都必须切除。如果诊断为外阴上皮内瘤样病变，适合做切除术。浸润性癌最好行肿瘤根治术（图99，100，101），向深部切除达深筋膜，另外切除正常皮肤边缘 > 1cm。如果肿瘤浸润深度 > 1cm，需要切除腹股沟淋巴结。如果肿瘤仅位于一侧，只需切除患侧淋巴结。如果肿瘤长在中央，需做两侧腹股沟淋巴结切除术。如果肿瘤不能切除，放化疗就被用做一线治疗方法，有时当肿瘤蔓延至接近切除边缘时，放疗就很必要。

并发症 并发症包括伤口血肿和淋巴结切除后导致腹股沟淋巴囊肿形成；这些通常与淋巴间断回流有关。淋巴管性水肿可能成为一种慢性并发症。

Cancer of the vulva

Incidence and aetiology Vulval carcinoma is an uncommon condition usually confined to older women and associated with underlying vulval conditions such as lichen sclerosus et atrophicus. There has, however, been a rise in incidence in younger women, associated with high-risk HPV types and smoking.

Pathology Carcinoma of the vulva (Fig. 98) is usually slow-growing and the vast majority are squamous cell tumours. Most of the lymphatics drain directly to the superficial and deep inguinal nodes and then to the iliac chain. Basal cell carcinoma and melanoma are rare.

Clinical features Usually presents with a lump or mass or ulceration and a history of pruritus.

Management All suspicious lesions must be biopsied. If vulval intra-epithelial neoplasia is diagnosed, excision may be appropriate. Invasive carcinoma is best managed by radical excision of the tumour (Figs 99, 100, 101), i.e. achieving deep clearance down to the underlying fascia, and an adequate skin margin of >1cm. Removal of the inguinofemoral lymph nodes is necessary if the depth of invasion of the tumour is >1mm. If the tumour is well lateralized only the nodes on that side need be removed. If the tumour is central, bilateral inguinofemoral lymphadenectomy is indicated.

Chemo-irradiation is used as first-line treatment if the tumour is not excisable and radiotherapy is sometimes necessary if the tumour extends close to the excision margins.

Complications Complications include wound haematoma and lymphocele formation at the groin as a consequence of node dissection; these usually resolve with intermittent drainage. Lymphoedema can be a chronic complication.

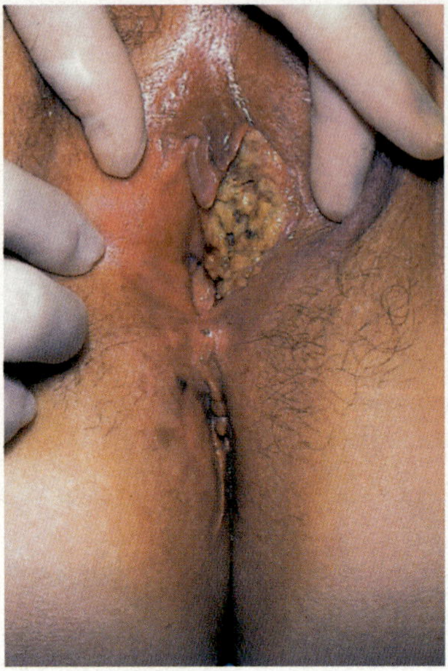

图 98 浸润性癌
Invasive carcinoma

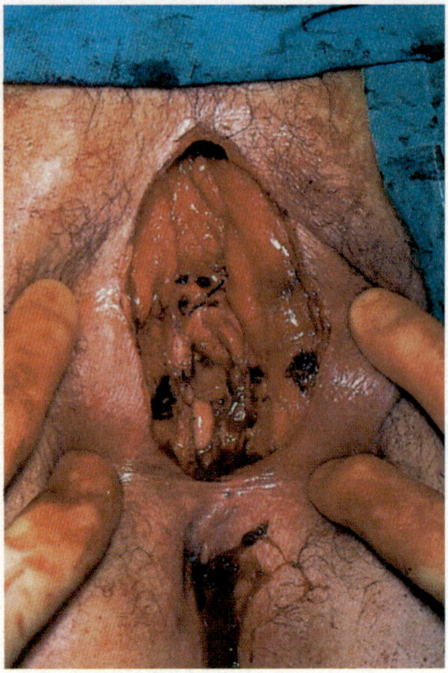

图 99 外阴切除
Excision of the vulva

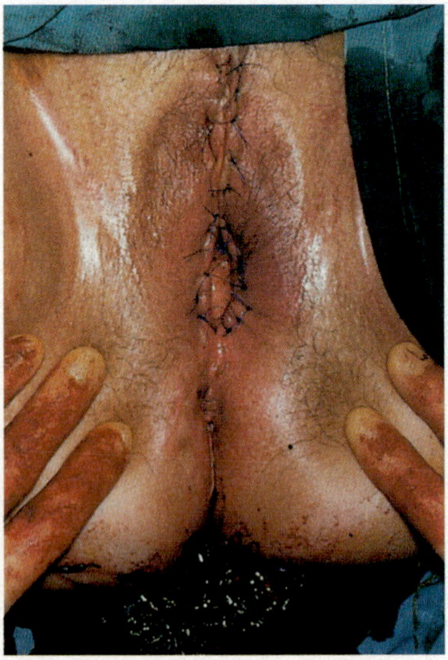

图 100 术后所见
Postoperative appearance

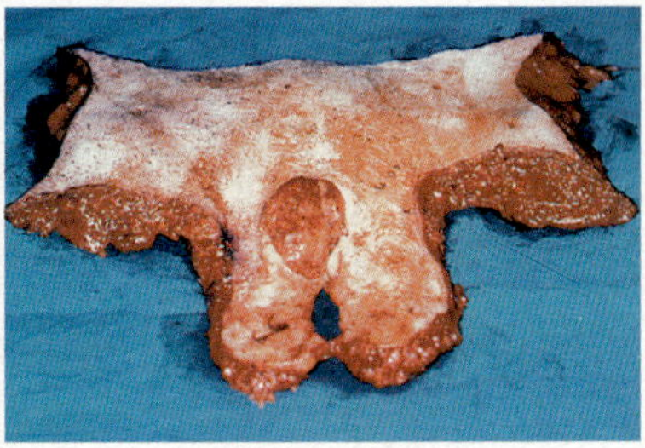

图 101 外阴癌手术标本
Surgical specimen of vulval carcinoma

阴道和宫颈良性病变、癌前病变及恶性疾病

正常宫颈

正常宫颈阴道部被覆复层鳞状上皮（图102），宫颈管腔被覆柱状上皮（图103），两者交界处称为鳞柱交界。鳞柱交界的位置可以变化，青春期、妊娠期和使用口服避孕药都可以引起宫颈管外翻，因此显现了更大区域的柱状上皮，肉眼见呈红色，称之为异位。

这一区域中间至原始鳞柱交界称为移行带。化生（一种细胞转化成另一种细胞）就在这一区域发生，如柱状细胞转化为成熟的鳞状上皮。

良性疾病

宫颈炎

某些细菌好感染宫颈柱状上皮，如沙眼衣原体和淋病奈瑟菌，导致宫颈炎外观。

宫颈肌瘤

呈带蒂生长或长在宫颈体内，可以生长成一定体积而充填阴道。

宫颈息肉

多起源于宫颈管内，带蒂，被覆宫颈管柱状上皮。体积大小相差很大，表面有鲜红色血管生长（图104）。宫颈内息肉表现为无症状或不规则阴道流血和/或性交后出血。治疗可用撕脱法。如为宽基底也以用结扎法。

13 Benign, premalignant and malignant conditions of the vagina and cervix

The normal cervix

The normal ectocervix is covered with stratified squamous epithelium (Fig. 102). The endocervical canal is lined by columnar epithelium (Fig. 103). The junction between these two types is known as the *squamocolumnar junction*.
The position of the squamocolumnar junction varies. Puberty, pregnancy and the use of the oral contraceptive pill cause eversion of the canal, thus displaying a greater area of columnar epithelium, which has a red appearance to the naked eye. This is termed *ectopy*.
The area medial to the original squamocolumnar junction is termed the transformation zone. It is in this area that metaplasia (the change of one cell type to another) takes place, i.e. columnar cells are transformed to mature squamous epithelium.

Benign conditions

Cervicitis

Certain bacteria preferentially infect columnar epithelium, e.g. *Chlamydia trachomatis* and *Neisseria gonorrhoeae*, giving rise to appearances described as cervicitis.

Cervical fibroids

These may be pedunculated or within the body of the cervix, perhaps growing to a size that fills the vagina.

Cervical polyps

These usually arise from the endocervix and are pedunculated with a covering of endocervical epithelium. They vary considerably in size and appear as bright red vascular growths (Fig. 104). Endocervical polyps may be symptomless or may present with irregular vaginal bleeding and/or postcoital bleeding. Treatment is by avulsion. If the base is broad it may require ligation.

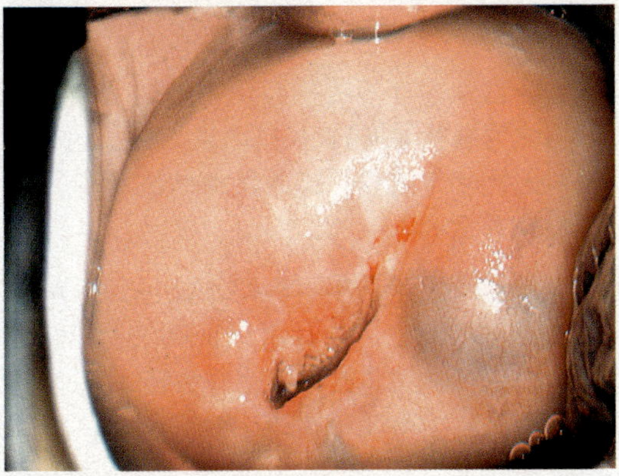

图 102　正常宫颈阴道镜图
Colpophotograph of a normal cervix

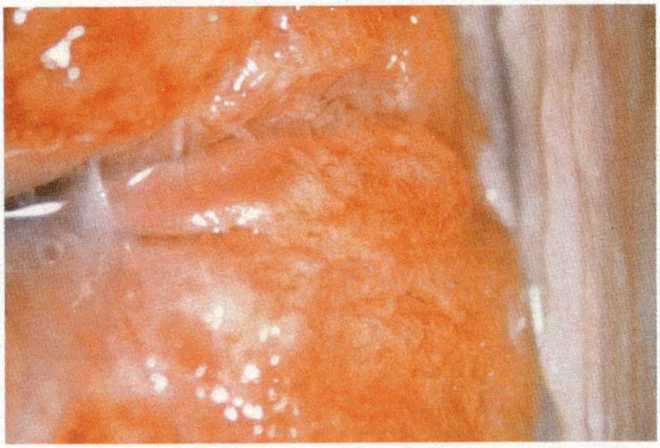

图 103　宫颈柱状上皮——高倍镜
Cervical columnar epithelium —— high power

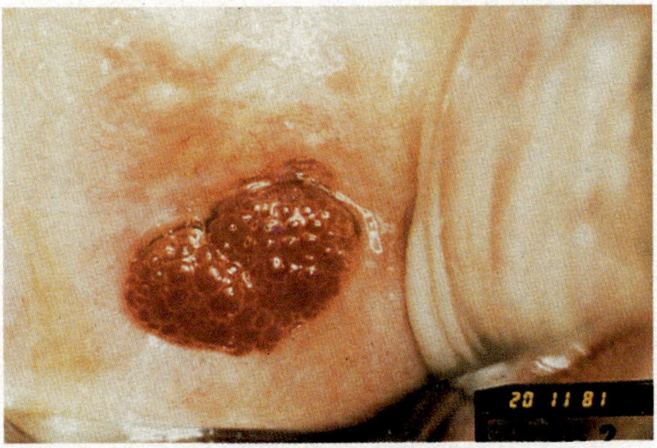

图 104　宫颈内息肉——阴道镜图
Endocervical polyp —— colpophotograph

癌前病变

在宫颈移行带区存在化生过程（细胞由柱状上皮转化为鳞状上皮）。某些因素如疣状病毒（HPV）可以干扰化生过程，结果使鳞状细胞变得不规则（即发育异常）。

临床特征

在宫颈癌前病变，肉眼不能见到异常，宫颈涂片筛查可以确定。涂片可以证明细胞核异常（图105），根据细胞的非典型程度分为轻、中、重度（图106）。核异常细胞明显表现为鳞状细胞，但表现出某些恶性特征：核增大，染色质增多，核边缘不规则。

检查

妇女应每隔三年进行宫颈涂片检查，如有两张交界性或肉眼可见的核异常涂片，或者一个中度的或者重度的核异型涂片，应行阴道镜检查。使用醋酸染色宫颈，不成熟的化生及核异常区域（图107）被染成白色（称为醋酸白）。白色区域的密度和其他特征包括*点状*（图108）、*镶嵌现象*（图109）以及*非典型血管形成*可以提示宫颈异常的程度。对宫颈异常区域进行活检或切除，以确定组织学诊断。

Premalignant conditions

In the transformation zone of the cervix there is an ongoing process of metaplasia (change of cell type from columnar to squamous epithelium). Interference with this normal process by factors such as wart virus (HPV) means that the resultant squamous cells are irregular (dysplastic).

Clinical features

Premalignant conditions of the cervix do not look abnormal to the naked eye. They are identified by cervical smear screening. The smear may demonstrate dyskaryotic cells (Fig. 105), graded as mild, moderate or severe (Fig. 106), depending on the degree of atypia. A dyskaryotic cell is clearly recognizable as a squamous cell but displays some of the features of malignancy: the nucleus is enlarged, the chromatin is increased and the nuclear borders are irregular.

Investigations

Women should have smears taken at 3-yearly intervals. Women should be referred for colposcopy after two borderline or visibly dyskaryotic smears, or one moderate or severely dyskaryotic smear.
Colposcopy is used to identify the lesion giving rise to the dyskaryotic cells exfoliated by the cervical smear. Using acetic acid to stain the cervix, areas of immature metaplasia and dysplasia (Fig. 107) are seen as white ('acetowhite'). The density of this whiteness together with other features, including *punctation* (Fig. 108), *mosaicism* (Fig. 109, p. 83), and atypical vessel formation, suggest the degree of abnormality present. The abnormal areas can be biopsied or excised to make a histological diagnosis.

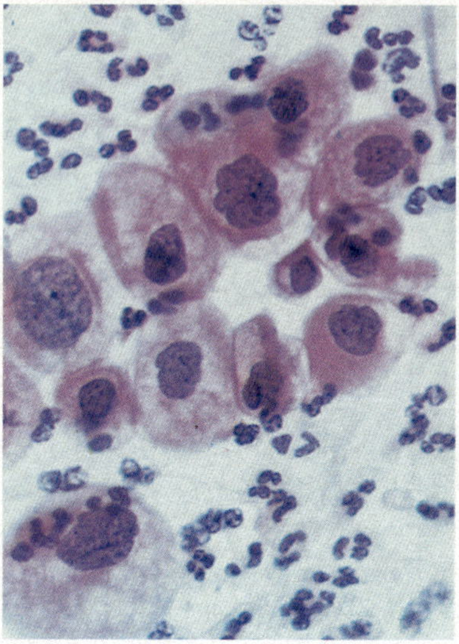

图 105　宫颈细胞学显示核异型
Cervical cytology showing dyskaryosis

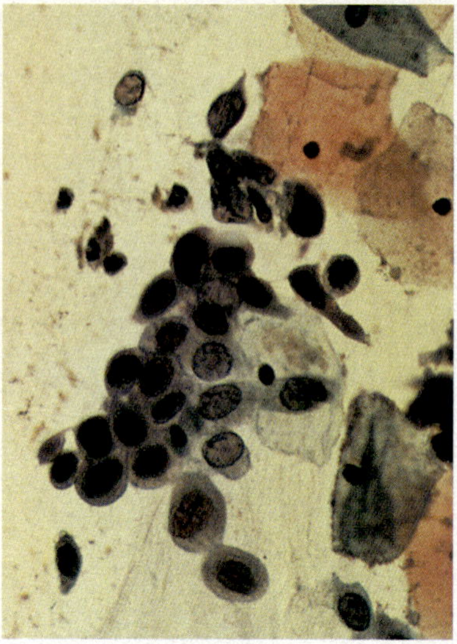

图 106　宫颈细胞学显示严重的核异型
Cervical cytology showing severe dyskaryosis

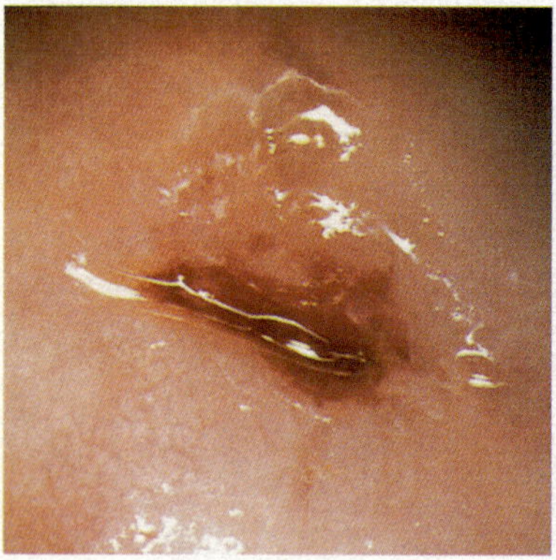

图 107　醋酸白改变
Acetowhite changes

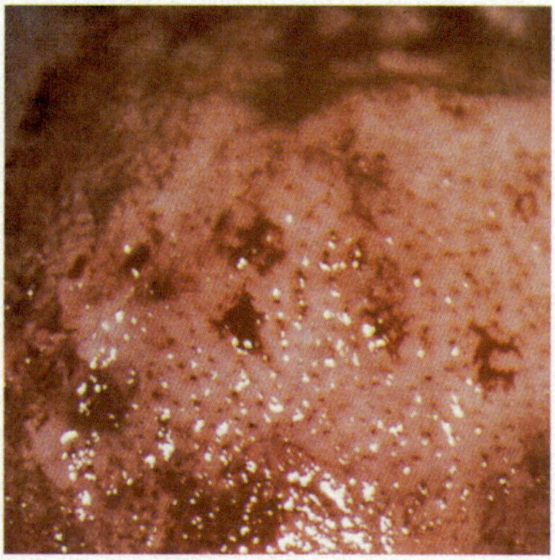

图 108　显著的点状改变
Marked punctation

分级

根据发育异常的程度，组织学可分为CIN（宫颈上皮内瘤变）Ⅰ、Ⅱ、Ⅲ。发育异常是组织学术语，用于描述上皮疾病（即部分上皮层被非典型细胞取代）（图 110）。

如不治疗，CIN 可能会发展成宫颈癌。

- *CIN Ⅰ*：上皮基底层上 1/3 被异型细胞取代。
- *CIN Ⅱ*：上皮基底层上 2/3 被异型细胞取代，且改变更加明显。
- *CIN Ⅲ*：上皮全层可见核异型（图 111，112）。

易感因素

高危型 HPV 如 16、18 和 32 型，以及吸烟是目前与 CIN 相关的主要因素。

治疗

CIN可以保守治疗，并规律随访直至宫颈异常病变消退。

CIN Ⅱ 和Ⅲ通常行宫颈环切除术。这能够在局麻下进行，并且因为能提供较好的组织病理标本，能够在第一次就诊时就完成（访问和治疗）。一旦获得活检标本就可以采用激光切除术和电烧术。如不能看到宫颈管内移行带的上界，宫颈锥形活检就很有必要了。

Grading

The histological findings are graded as CIN (cervical intraepithelial neoplasia) I, II and III, depending on the degree of dysplasia. Dysplasia is a histological term used to describe a lesion in which part of the thickness of the epithelium is replaced by atypical cells (Fig. 110).

If untreated, CIN may progress to cervical cancer.

- *CIN I* : the atypia is confined to the basal one-third of the epithelium.
- *CIN II* : the basal two-thirds are involved and the changes are more marked.
- *CIN III*: nuclear abnormalities are present throughout the whole thickness of the epithelium (Figs 111, 112).

Predisposing factors

High-risk HPV types, i.e. 16, 18 and 32, and smoking are the major factors currently associated with CIN.

Management

CIN can be managed conservatively with regular follow-up until the abnormality regresses.

CIN II and III are usually treated by loop excision. This can be performed under local anaesthetic and as it provides a good histopathology specimen, can be done at the first visit (see and treat). Laser ablation and electrical cauterization can be used once a biopsy specimen has been obtained. Cone biopsy is necessary if the upper limit of the transformation zone cannot be visualized in the canal.

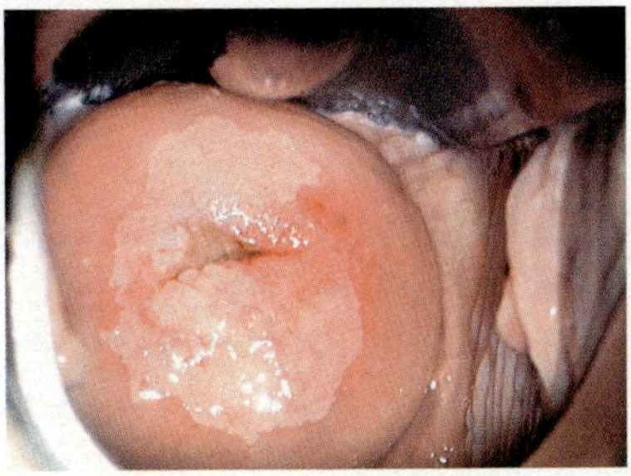

图 109　红色的镶嵌现象
Florid mosaicism

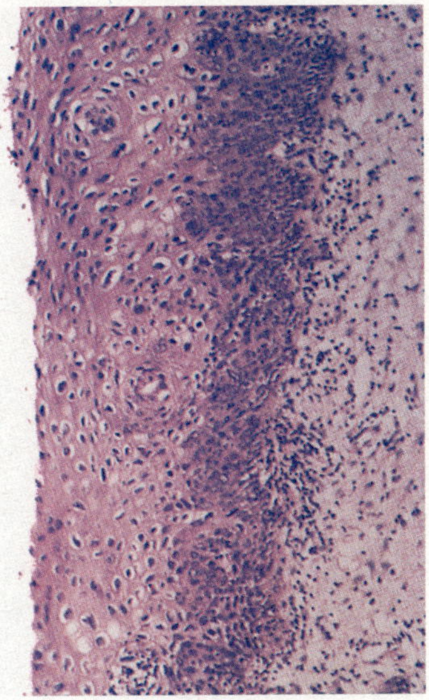

图 110　人乳头瘤病毒和 CIN
Human papilloma virus and CIN

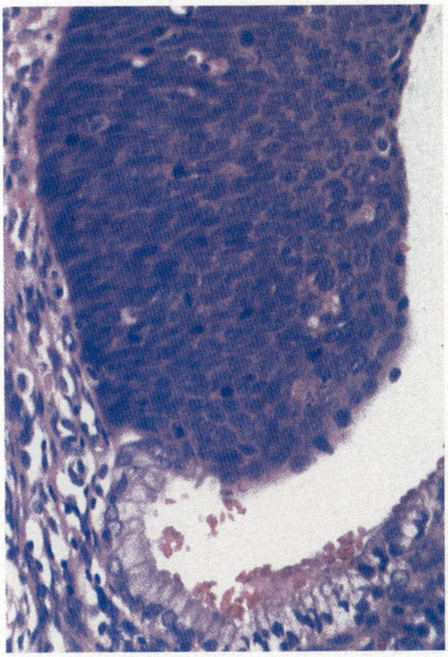

图 111　CINIII 和正常宫颈内膜
CIN III and normal endocervix

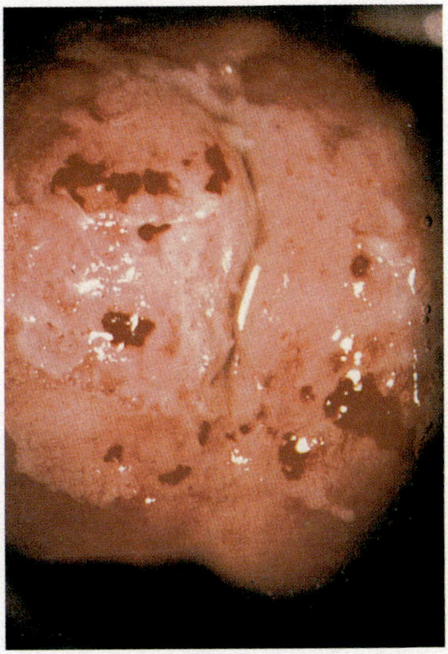

图 112　CINIII 肉眼所见
Macroscopic view of CIN III

宫颈癌

发病率

目前在英格兰和威尔士每年有 2700 人患宫颈癌，1200人死于该病。由于英国有效的国民健康保险制度的宫颈筛查计划，发病率和死亡率正在下降。

病因

宫颈癌在发展中国家较常见，在低水平社会经济群体中其发病率更高，宫颈癌本质上是一种性传播疾病。

宫颈癌易感因素很多，目前疣病毒与宫颈癌密切相关，吸烟对宫颈癌也有作用。

分期

因为世界上绝大多数病人仅通过放疗治疗，宫颈癌按照临床（麻醉下检查、宫颈活检、宫腔镜和膀胱镜检查）分期。在发达国家更多地使用MRI扫描作为分期工具。

Ⅰ期

- 1a：间质浸润深度≤ 5mm，两侧宽度≤ 7mm
- 1b：临床可见癌灶局限于宫颈

  1b1：≤ 4cm

  1b2：＞ 4 cm

Ⅱ期

癌灶超出宫颈但未达盆壁，癌灶累及阴道但未达阴道下 1/3。

Ⅲ期

癌灶达盆壁，阴道浸润已达下1/3。所有病例有肾盂积水或一个无功能肾，除非它们是由其他原因引起。

Ⅳ期

癌灶超出真骨盆或临床上累及膀胱或直肠黏膜（图114）。

Carcinoma of the cervix

Incidence

In England and Wales there are currently 2700 cases of cervical cancer per year and 1200 deaths from the disease. Incidence and mortality are falling because of the effectiveness of the NHS cervical screening programme in the UK.

Aetiology

Carcinoma of the cervix is more frequently seen in developing countries and its incidence is higher in lower socioeconomic groups. Cancer of the cervix is essentially a sexually transmitted disease.

A number of factors may predispose to cervical cancer. Presently the wart virus has the strongest association. Smoking may also have a role.

Staging

Cancer of the cervix is staged clinically (by examination under anaesthesia, cervical biopsy, hysteroscopy and cystoscopy) because worldwide most patients will be treated only with radiotherapy. In developed countries MRI scanning is used increasingly as a staging tool.

Stage I

- 1a: Stromal invasion of ⩽ 5 mm, extension ⩽ 5 mm with lateral extension of ⩽ 7 mm
- 1b: Clinically visible lesions limited to the cervix -
  1b1 ⩽ 4 cm
  1b2 > 4 cm

Stage II

The carcinoma extends beyond the cervix but has not extended onto the pelvic side wall. The carcinoma involves the vagina but not as far as the lower one-third.

Stage III

Carcinoma extends to the pelvic side wall. The lower one-third of the vagina may be involved. All cases with a hydronephrosis or a non-functioning kidney, unless they are known to be due to another cause.

Stage IV

Carcinoma has extended beyond the true pelvis or has clinically involved the mucosa of the bladder or rectum (Fig. 114).

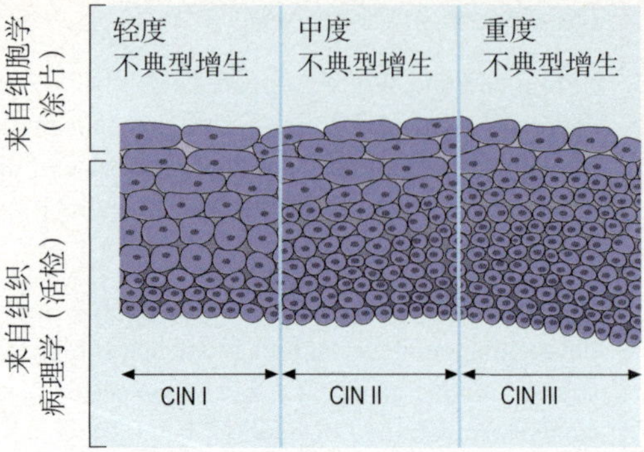

图 113 CIN 分级系统
The CIN grading system

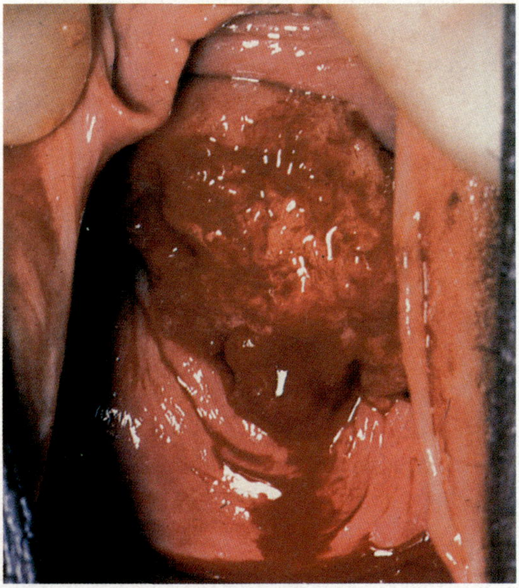

图 114 宫颈浸润癌
Frank invasive carcinoma of the cervix

病理　90% 以上的宫颈癌是鳞癌，起源于宫颈移行带区。其余为腺癌。宫颈癌通过直接扩散或淋巴道转移。

临床特征　患者可以表现为阴道流血，特别是性生活后出血。可能有阴道排液。早期癌可无症状，在筛查时发现。

检查　一旦组织学诊断确定后，需行麻醉下检查进行分期。通常应做胸片、静脉肾盂造影、常规生化和血液检查。CT 扫描对晚期癌和复发癌有帮助。

处理　镜下浸润癌通常建议行子宫切除术。对要求保留生育功能的年轻女性可考虑行宫颈锥切术。Ⅰb或Ⅱa期宫颈癌可用放疗或根治性Wertheim子宫切除术（切除全子宫、双输卵管、阴道上1/3、宫旁组织和盆腔淋巴结）。Wertheim 子宫切除术是要求保留卵巢功能、避免因放疗引起阴道狭窄和胃肠道副作用的年轻女性的选择性治疗方法。根治性宫颈切除术（切除宫颈但不包括宫体——图 115）正被评估用于希望保留生育功能的某些早期癌患者。放疗和根治性手术对早期癌的治疗效果是相似的，5年生存率均超过 80%。淋巴结有转移者 5 年生存率将减半。晚期癌普遍采用放疗，配合以铂类为主的化疗。

阴道癌

极少见，高发年龄为 60 ~ 70 岁，表现症状为阴道流血或脓性白带。治疗取决于组织学分型、临床分期和患者健康状况。可采用手术、放疗和手术+放疗的联合治疗。

Pathology

Up to 90% of cervical cancers are squamous cell tumours originating in the transformation zone. Adenocarcinomas account for the remainder of cases. Cervical cancer spreads by direct extension or via the lymphatics.

Clinical features

Patients may present with vaginal bleeding, particularly after intercourse. There may be vaginal discharge. Early lesions may be symptomless and are detected by screening.

Investigations

Once the diagnosis is confirmed histologically an EUA is necessary for staging. Chest X-ray, IVP and routine biochemical and haematological investigations are usually required. CT scan is helpful in advanced and recurrent disease.

Management

Hysterectomy is usually advised for microinvasive disease. Cone biopsy may be considered in a young woman desiring children. Stage Ib or IIa cervical cancer can be treated by either radiotherapy or radical Wertheim's hysterectomy (removal of the uterus, fallopian tubes, upper one-third of the vagina, parametrium and pelvic lymph nodes). Wertheim's hysterectomy is the treatment of choice in younger women who wish to retain ovarian function and avoid vaginal stenosis and gastrointestinal side effects, which may be caused by radiotherapy. Radical trachelectomy (the removal of the cervix but not the uterine body - Fig. 115) is being evaluated as a fertility-sparing treatment for some women with early-stage disease. The results of radiotherapy and radical surgery in early stage disease are similar, both having 5-year survival rates in excess of 80%. The finding of tumour in lymph nodes will halve this survival rate. Radiotherapy is commonly used in more advanced diseases in combination with platinum-based chemotherapy.

Carcinoma of the vagina

Rare and tends to occur mainly in the 6th and 7th decades. Presenting symptoms are vaginal bleeding or a purulent discharge. Treatment of the condition is determined by histology, staging and the health of the patient. Surgery, radiotherapy and a combination of both have been used.

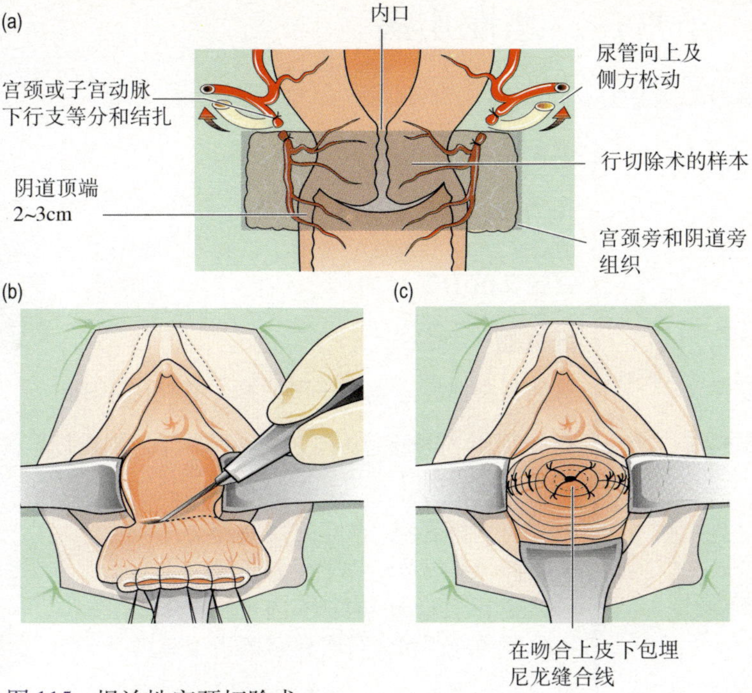

图 115　根治性宫颈切除术
Radical trachelectomy

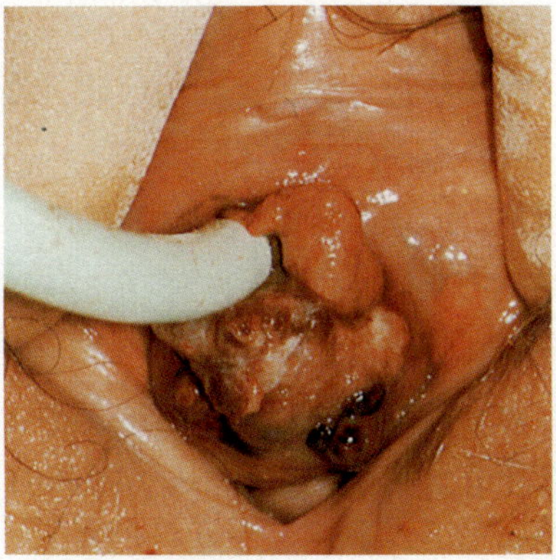

图 116　阴道癌
Vaginal carcinoma

14 子宫良、恶性疾病

先天畸形

先天性无子宫很少见，这样的患者可能有痕迹阴道。先天畸形包括从弓形子宫到完全的双子宫和双宫颈（图 117，118）。

纤维瘤

定义

普通平滑肌肿瘤也称平滑肌瘤，其病因不清。

发病率

在高加索人种中 30 岁以上妇女纤维瘤发生率在 20% 以上。

分类

- *浆膜下纤维瘤*：从子宫腹膜面突出
- *肌壁间纤维瘤*：位于子宫肌壁内
- *黏膜下纤维瘤*：向宫腔内侵及
- *带蒂的纤维瘤*：可来自浆膜下或黏膜下

病理

纤维瘤来自生育期平滑肌细胞，在雌激素刺激下体积增加。

临床特征

绝大多数纤维瘤无症状。也可引起痛经、腹胀和压迫症状（如尿频）。通常无疼痛，除非发生纤维瘤变性或蒂扭转。

腹部检查可触及盆腔内包块，盆腔检查可证实包块且其表面不规则。

检查

包括超声、麻醉下检查、宫腔镜，如有不规则流血应做子宫内膜活检。

处理

可以保守治疗或手术治疗（图 119）。

并发症

纤维瘤血供少，可能会变性（玻璃样变、囊性变、红色变、肉瘤变）、钙化（图 120）和/或坏死。纤维瘤可继发感染、扭转，但很少转移。

14 Benign and malignant conditions of the uterus

Congenital anomalies

Congenital absence of the uterus is rare, and in such cases a rudimentary vagina may be present. Congenital anomalies range from an arcuate uterus to a complete duplication of the uterus and cervix (Figs 117, 118).

Fibroids

Definition
Common smooth muscle tumours also known as leiomyomata. Aetiology unknown.

Incidence
Fibroids occur in more than 20% of Caucasian women over 30 years.

Classification
- *Subserous*: project from the peritoneal surface of the uterus
- *Intramural*: lie within the uterine wall
- *Submucous*: encroach on the uterine cavity
- *Pedunculated*: can arise from subserous or submucous

Pathology
Fibroids arise from smooth muscle cells during reproductive life and can increase in size in response to oestrogen.

Clinical features
The majority of fibroids are symptomless. They may cause menorrhagia, abdominal distension and pressure symptoms such as urinary frequency. Pain is unusual unless there is red degeneration or torsion of a pedunculated fibroid.

Abdominal examination may reveal a palpable mass arising from the pelvis. Pelvic examination will confirm this and the outline may be irregular.

Investigations
These include ultrasonography, EUA, hysteroscopy and endometrial biopsy if abnormal bleeding.

Management
Treatment can either be conservative or surgical (Fig. 119).

Complications
The poor vascularity of fibroids encourages degeneration (hyaline, cystic, red, sarcomatous), calcification (Fig. 120) and/or necrosis. Fibroids can also become infected, tort and rarely metastasize.

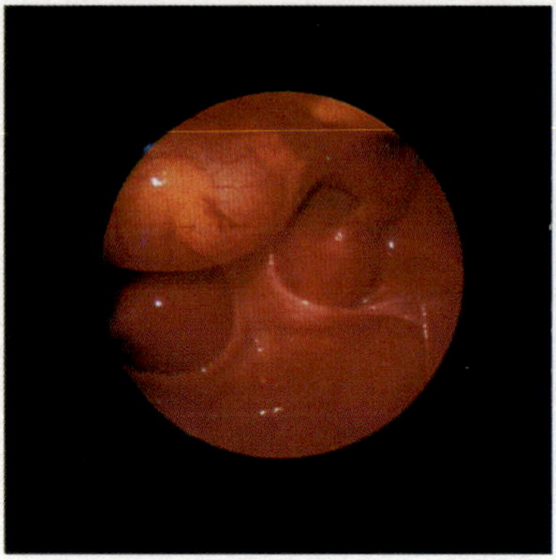

图 117 腹腔镜下见双角子宫
Laparoscopic view of bicornuate uterus

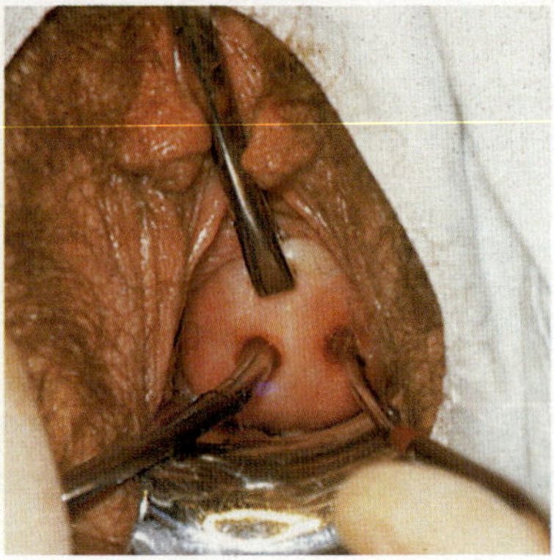

图 118 双宫颈，每个宫颈口插入一个扩棒
A double cervix with a dilator in each os

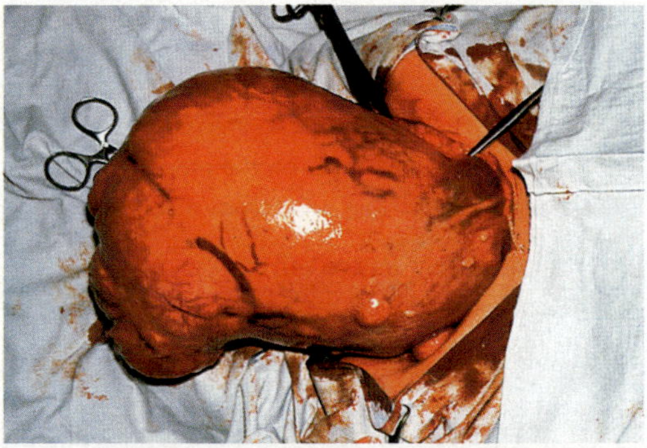

图 119 增大的子宫纤维瘤——手术标本
Enlarged fibroid uterus — operative specimen

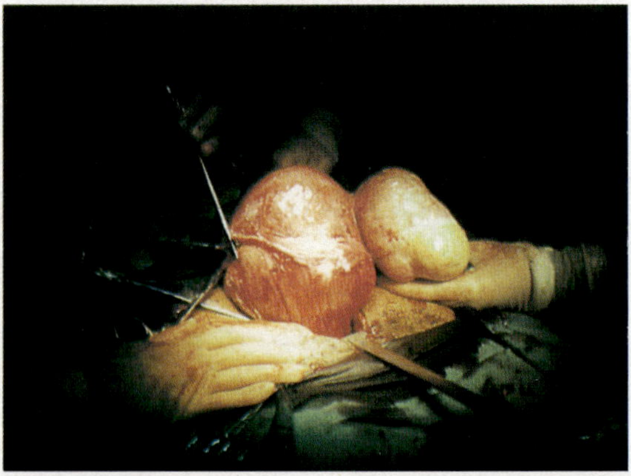

图 120 生长于左侧宫底的带蒂的纤维瘤
Enlarged uterus with a pedunculated fibroid arising from the left lateral fundus

子宫体癌

分类

子宫体癌绝大多数为腺癌（图 121），分期如下：

I 期：癌局限于宫体。
II 期：癌累及宫体及宫颈。
III 期：癌超出子宫，但未超出真骨盆。
IV 期：超出真骨盆或累及膀胱、直肠。

病因

子宫内膜癌绝大多数发生在绝经后妇女和长期接受雌激素刺激的女性，如未产妇、延迟绝经、肥胖和多囊卵巢综合征者，内膜增生是其前兆。

临床特征

内膜癌的典型表现为绝经后阴道流血，因此需要检查。如无易感因素（如多囊卵巢综合征），40 多岁以下的年轻女性很少发病。

腹部和盆腔检查包括宫颈涂片（所有病人都应检查）。阴式超声也有助于诊断（内膜增厚 > 5mm 是可疑的）。内膜活检和/或宫腔镜检查可在门诊进行（图 122），如不能进行，可采用全麻。

检查

经腹全子宫 + 双侧卵巢输卵管切除术在分期手术中进行，包括采集腹腔冲洗液。子宫内膜癌行淋巴结切除术的作用尚待评估。辅助放疗通常用于晚期癌和癌灶侵及超过子宫内膜外 1/2，以减少局部复发的风险。

处理

影响子宫内膜癌生存率的因素有：确诊时年龄、疾病分期、病理分型、癌分化程度和侵及肌层的深度。

Uterine cancer

Classification

The majority of lesions are adenocarcinoma (Fig. 121), and the staging is as follows:

Stage I: confined to the body of the uterus.
Stage II: involves the body and the cervix.
Stage III: extends beyond uterus but not beyond the true pelvis.
Stage IV: extends outside true pelvis or involves bladder or rectum.

Aetiology

Endometrial cancer occurs mostly in postmenopausal women and women who have had prolonged exposure to oestrogen stimulation, i.e. nulliparous women, late menopause, obese women and women with polycystic ovaries. Hyperplasia is a precursor.

Clinical features

Postmenopausal bleeding is the classic presentation for endometrial carcinoma and therefore requires investigation. It is rare in women under the age of 40, unless there are predisposing factors, e.g. PCO.

Clinical features

Abdominal and pelvic examinations, including a cervical smear, should be carried out in all cases. Transvaginal ultrasound scanning may be helpful in identifying changes (>5 mm endometrial thickening is suspicious). Endometrial sampling and/or hysteroscopy (Fig. 122) can be performed in the outpatient clinic or, if that is not possible, under general anaesthetic.

Investigations

A total abdominal hysterectomy and bilateral salpingo-oophorectomy is performed during a staging operation which involves taking peritoneal washings. The role of lymphadenectomy in endometrial cancer is under evaluation. Adjuvant radiotherapy is sometimes used for high-grade lesions and cancers that involve the outer half of the endometrium to reduce the risk of local or regional recurrence.

Management

Factors influencing survival endometrial carcinoma are age at diagnosis, stage of disease, pathological type and degree of differentiation of the lesion and the depth of myometrial invasion.

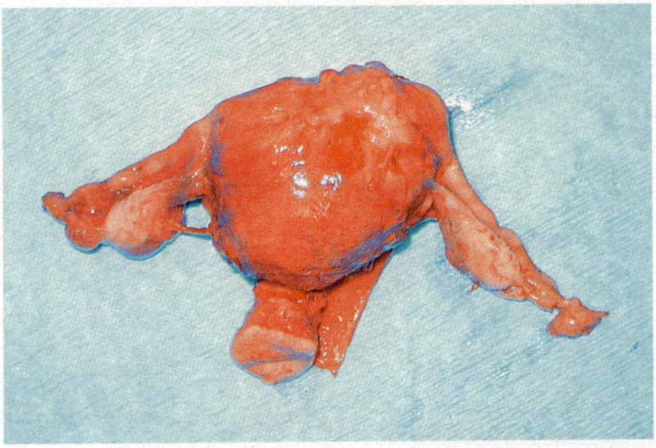

图 121　通过浆膜扩散的子宫内膜癌手术标本
Surgical specimen of an endometrial cancer spreading through the serosa

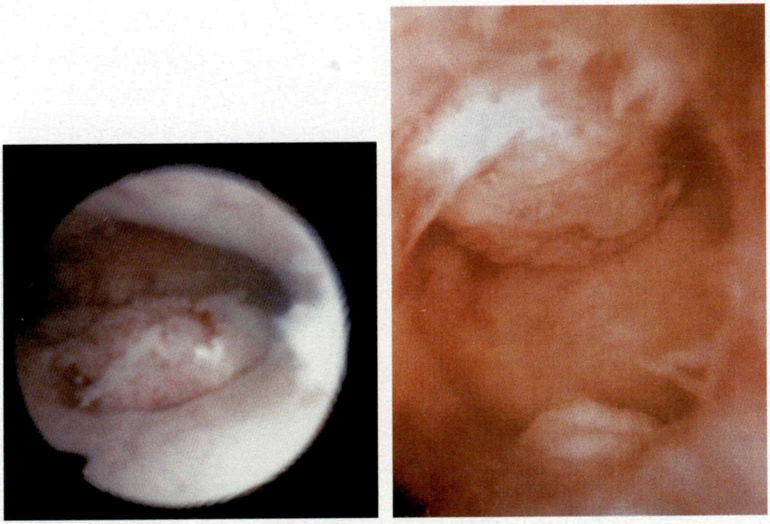

图 122　内膜癌宫腔镜图像
Hysteroscopic views of endometrial carcinoma

输卵管良、恶性疾病

卵子从卵泡释放后输卵管伞拾卵，输卵管内膜纤毛运输卵子到受精部位，精子被输卵管子宫末端的纤毛运送至受精处。

输卵管感染

输卵管可以因感染（或外伤后炎症）而形成输卵管阻塞，形成输卵管脓肿或输卵管积水。

临床特征

输卵管感染可以表现为急性腹痛，特别是如果脓肿已形成。输卵管积水可以是无症状的。

检查

腹腔镜对于探查输卵管腹膜面很有帮助。可在输卵管表面特别是伞部见到渗出液。如输卵管伞端呈棒状改变，则表明为慢性损害。还可以见到新鲜和陈旧的粘连灶。输卵管积水可以表现为输卵管肿大但并不是活动性感染。如果无急性感染，可以通过宫颈注入染色剂。若无输卵管阻塞可见染色剂填充输卵管，并可以自由流至腹腔。子宫输卵管造影术是一项有用的诊断技术。

治疗

急性感染应该被合理治疗。由于输卵管损害引起的不孕症可以通过输卵管手术或体外受精来解决输卵管梗阻。

输卵管癌

原发性输卵管癌较罕见（图124），更常见的为来自邻近器官的转移癌。典型症状是水性、血性阴道排液。通过检查可能触及附件包块。卵巢肿瘤标记物CA125值通常升高。治疗是经腹全子宫切除术及双卵巢输卵管切除术，术后同卵巢癌一样辅以化疗。

Benign and malignant conditions of the fallopian tubes

15

The fimbriae of the fallopian tubes pick up the ovum after it is released from the follicle and the cilia of the endosalpinx transport it to the site of fertilization. Sperm are carried there by the cilia from the uterine end of the tube.

Tubal infection

The tubes can become blocked by infection (or inflammation following trauma). The result of this can be tubal abscess or hydrosalpinx (Fig. 123).

Clinical features

Tubal infection may present with pain of an acute abdomen, especially if an abscess has formed. A hydrosalpinx may be symptomless.

Investigations

Laparoscopy is useful for inspection of the peritoneal aspect of the tubes. Exudate may be seen over the tubes, especially at the fimbriae. If the fimbriae are clubbed, this indicates chronic damage. Fresh and old adhesions may be seen. A hydrosalpinx will be visualized as a swollen tube but not actively infected. In the absence of acute infection, dye can be injected through the cervix. If there is no tubal blockage, filling of the tubes and free spill into the peritoneal cavity can be seen. Hysterosalpingography is a useful investigative technique.

Management

Acute infection should be treated appropriately. Infertility due to tubal damage can be treated by tubal surgery or in vitro fertilization to overcome tubal blockage.

Cancer of the fallopian tube

Primary cancer of the fallopian tube (Fig.124) is rare; secondary disease from adjacent structures is more common. The symptoms are classically a watery, bloody vaginal discharge. On examination, an adnexal mass may be felt. The ovarian tumour marker CA125 is often raised. The treatment is total abdominal hysterectomy and bilateral oophorectomy followed by chemotherapy as for ovarian cancer.

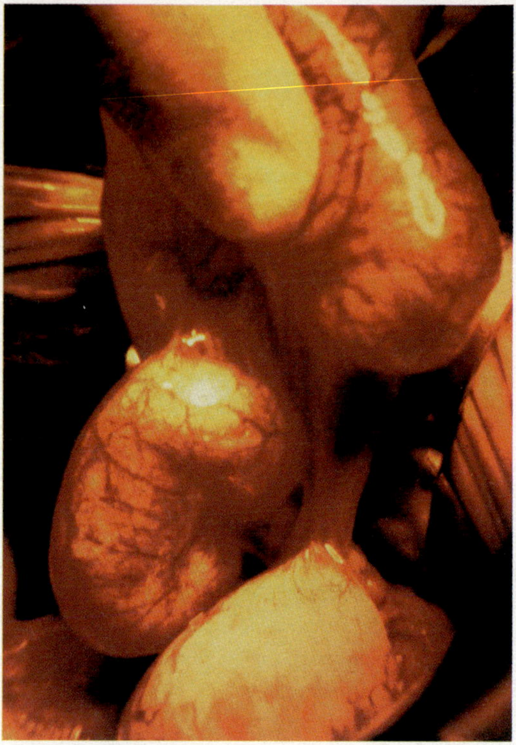

图 123 输卵管积水
Hydrosalpinx

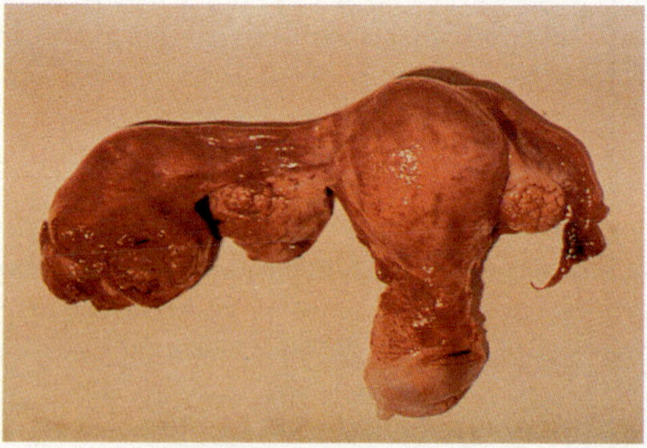

图 124 输卵管癌
Carcinoma of the fallopian tube

卵巢囊肿可以是生理性的、良性的（图125）或恶性的。卵巢病理可以出现以下症状:

- 卵巢增大会引起膀胱、直肠压迫症状或引起腹胀
- 是否有卵巢/囊肿扭转、出血或破裂
- 可影响激素生成

生理性囊肿（增大扩张的囊肿）

临床分型

卵泡囊肿　由没能破裂的卵泡增大引起。它们可能与无排卵周期、避孕药物、多囊卵巢综合征有关，通常无症状而自然消退。

黄体囊肿　能够引起闭经，随后有明显的阴道流血。自然消退很常见，但是腹腔内出血会引起明显疼痛。

子宫内膜异位症　由沉积在卵巢表面的子宫内膜内陷形成。

多囊卵巢　增大（图126），伴多个被膜下小卵泡。

卵巢肿瘤——良性和恶性

发病率

卵巢良性肿瘤较常见。在英国卵巢癌发病率为14∶100 000。卵巢癌发病率随年龄增大而升高，60岁为发病高峰。

临床表现

卵巢癌通常无症状或无特异性症状（如消化不良）。老年女性应当警惕恶性肿瘤发生的可能，特别是卵巢呈固定的、双侧发病、生长迅速，或与腹水有关时。超声下实性的或混合性囊肿及实性表面的囊肿也能提示卵巢癌。在晚期卵巢癌可表现双下肢静脉梗死、疼痛和可触及锁骨上淋巴结肿大。

16 Benign and malignant conditions of the ovary

Ovarian cysts may be physiological, benign (Fig. 125) or malignant tumours. Ovarian pathology may give rise to symptoms:

- when ovarian enlargement causes pressure on the bladder or rectum or abdominal distension
- if the ovary/cyst torts, bleeds or ruptures
- should hormonal production be affected

Physiological cysts (distension cysts)

Clinical types

Follicular cysts Due to enlargement of follicles which fail to rupture. They may be associated with anovulatory cycles, fertility drugs and PCOs. Usually symptomless and resolve spontaneously.

Corpus luteum cysts Can cause amenorrhoea followed by heavy vaginal bleeding. Spontaneous resolution is the norm but intra-abdominal bleeding may cause significant pain.

Endometriomas Result from invagination of endometrial deposits on the surface of the ovary.

Polycystic ovaries Enlarged (Fig. 126), with numerous small subcapsular follicular cysts.

Ovarian tumours — benign and malignant

Incidence

Benign tumours of the ovary are common. Ovarian cancer has an incidence of 14:100 000 women in the UK. The incidence of ovarian cancer increases with age, with the peak incidence in the sixties.

Clinical features

Ovarian cancer is often either symptomless or associated with non-specific symptoms such as dyspepsia. A malignant tumour should be suspected in older women, especially if it is fixed, bilateral, rapid-growing or associated with ascites. A solid, or a mixed cystic and solid appearance on ultrasound scanning is also suggestive. In advanced disease there may be venous obstruction of the legs, pain and palpable supraclavicular lymphadenopathy.

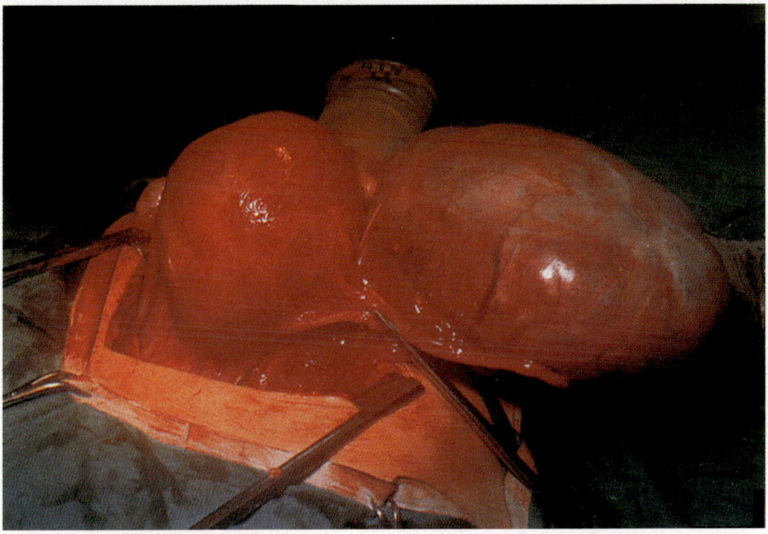

图 125　大的良性卵巢囊肿
Large benign ovarian cyst

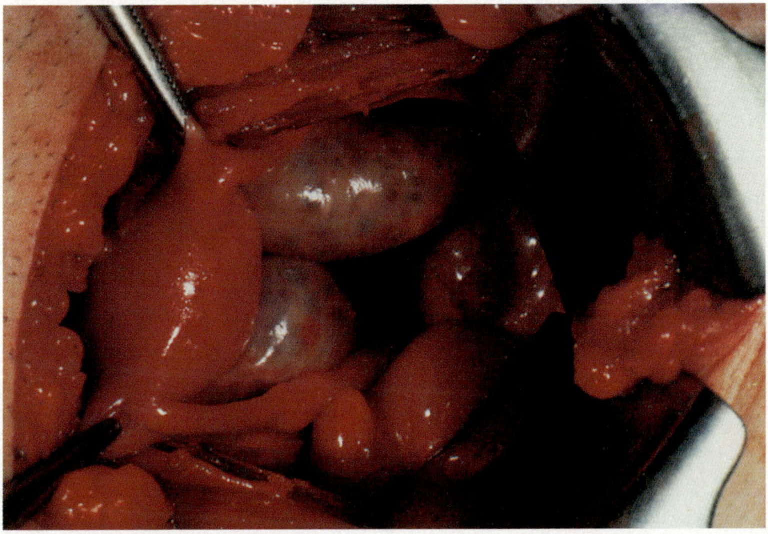

图 126　“Kissing”多囊卵巢
'Kissing' polycystic ovaries

分类

卵巢肿瘤可以根据以下细胞种类分类：

- 上皮性
- 生殖细胞
- 性索间质

乳腺、胃、大肠和子宫的原发性肿瘤也可在卵巢上产生继发性病灶（Krukenberg；图 127）。

上皮来源的肿瘤

大约90%卵巢癌来源于上皮组织。这些肿瘤进一步分为：

- *浆液性*，如浆液性囊腺瘤（良性）、浆液性囊腺癌（恶性，图 128）。
- *黏液性*，如黏液性囊腺瘤、黏液性囊腺癌。
- *子宫内膜样癌*
- *Brenner 瘤*
- *透明细胞瘤*

上皮性卵巢肿瘤可以是良性、交界性或恶性的。卵巢恶性肿瘤大多是腺癌。

生殖细胞来源的肿瘤

卵巢的生殖细胞是全能细胞（例如能分化为多种组织）。生殖细胞来源的肿瘤可能含有各种组织，包括牙齿、骨骼、软骨组织、肌肉、甲状腺和神经组织。最常见的生殖细胞来源的肿瘤是良性囊性畸胎瘤（皮样囊肿，图 129）。这些肿瘤是年轻女性最常见的肿瘤。在 10% ~ 20% 病例中是双侧发病的。

性索间质来源的肿瘤

性索肿瘤是罕见的。颗粒细胞瘤和卵泡膜细胞瘤分泌雌激素，因而使尚未月经来潮的女孩发生青春期性早熟，还可引起子宫内膜增生和老年妇女绝经后出血。50%以上的颗粒细胞瘤是恶性的；绝大多数的卵泡膜细胞瘤是良性的。支持-间质细胞瘤可分泌雄激素，并因此导致进行性女性男性化。

Classification Ovarian tumours can be derived from the following cell types:

- surface epithelium
- germ cells
- gonadal stroma

Secondary deposits from primary tumours of the breast, stomach, large bowel and uterus may also occur in the ovaries (Krukenberg tumours; Fig. 127).

Tumours derived from surface epithelium

About 90% of ovarian tumours originate from the surface epithelium. These are further subdivided into:

- *Serous*, e.g. serous cystadenoma (benign), serous cystadenocarcinoma (malignant, Fig. 128)
- *Mucinous*, e.g. mucinous cystadenoma, mucinous cystadenocarcinoma
- *Endometrioid*
- *Brenner tumours*
- *Clear cell tumours*

Epithelial ovarian tumours can be benign, of borderline malignancy, or frankly malignant. The malignant forms are collectively known as adenocarcinoma of the ovary.

Tumours derived from germ cells

The germ cells of the ovary are totipotent (i.e. can give rise to various types of tissues). Tumours of germ cells can contain a variety of tissues including teeth, bone, cartilage, muscle, thyroid and nervous tissue. The most common germ cell tumour is the benign cystic teratoma (dermoid cyst, Fig. 129). These are the most common tumours in young women. They are bilateral in 10%~20% of cases.

Tumours derived from gonadal stroma

Sex cord tumours are rare. Granulosa cell tumours and thecomas secrete oestrogens and can therefore cause precocious puberty in premenarchal girls, and endometrial hyperplasia and postmenopausal bleeding in older women. More than 50% of granulosa cell tumours are malignant; the vast majority of thecomas are benign. Sertoli-Leydig tumours may secrete androgens and can therefore cause progressive virilization.

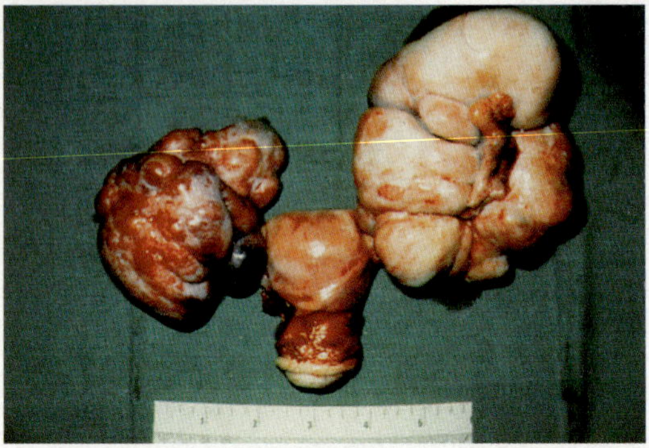

图 127　双侧 Krukenberg 瘤
Bilateral Krukenberg tumours

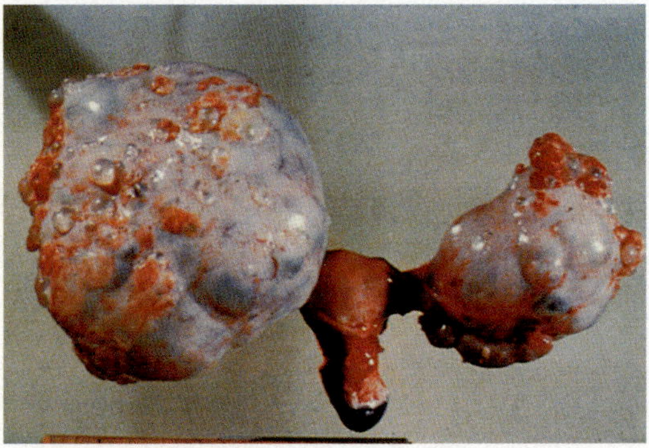

图 128　严重的囊腺瘤
Serous cystadenocarcinoma

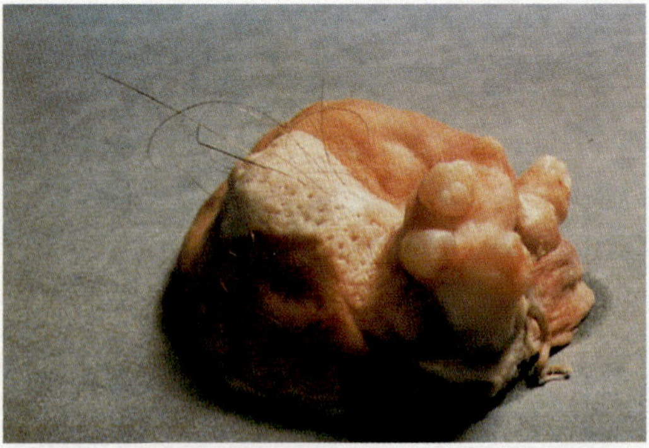

图 129　良性囊性畸胎瘤
Benign cystic teratoma

处理

手术之前，应评估卵巢癌的风险，以防止无经验的术者遇到卵巢癌（图 130， 131）。

卵巢癌

应对卵巢癌做充分的术前评估，并进行全面检查包括乳房和淋巴结。手术前超声检查和血清肿瘤标记物 CA125 检测可排除/减少恶变的机会，通常采用腹腔镜下囊肿/卵巢切除术。剖腹探查术的目的包括：适当的临床分期和切除所有可见肿瘤（图132，133）。

分期需要通过垂直切口切开后做全腹腔彻底探查。需要进行腹膜冲洗，并且下列范围应切除或活检：包括壁层腹膜，大网膜、子宫和对侧卵巢、肠管和肠系膜、膈肌和盆腔及主动脉旁淋巴结。

手术治疗

绝大多数卵巢癌手术目的是进行肿瘤细胞减灭术，随后进行术后化疗。

预后

原发性卵巢癌 5 年生存率如下： Ⅰa 85%， Ⅰb ~ Ⅱa 40%， Ⅱb 25%， Ⅱc ~ Ⅲ 15%， Ⅳ < 5%。在近 30 年卵巢癌预后变化很小，因为妇女始终在疾病的晚期就诊。

如果有可能在疾病的早期就发现，有效的筛查就很有价值。超声检查和各种肿瘤标记物（如 CA125）目前正被使用。筛查或预防性卵巢切除适用于那些具有卵巢癌高风险性的女性，如有较强和确定的家族史（2个或2个以上一级亲属患卵巢癌）或存在 BRCA1 或 BRCA2 基因突变者。

Management

Before embarking upon surgery, the risk of malignancy must be assessed to prevent inexperienced operators encountering ovarian cancer (Figs 130, 131).

Ovarian cancer

An adequate preoperative assessment should be made, with a general examination including the breasts and lymph nodes. With preoperative ultrasound and measurement of the serum tumour marker CA125 to exclude/reduce the chances of malignancy, laparoscopic removal of the cyst/ovary is often employed. Laparotomy aims include: adequate staging and removal of all visible tumour deposits (Figs 132, 133).

Staging requires thorough inspection of the whole abdominal cavity through a vertical incision. Peritoneal washings are taken and the following are either removed or biopsied: parietal peritoneum, omentum, uterus and other ovary, bowel and mesentery, diaphragm, and pelvic and para-aortic lymph nodes.

Surgical measures

In most cases of ovarian cancer the aim is cystoreductive surgery followed by chemotherapy.

Prognosis

The 5-year survival rates for primary ovarian cancer are as follows: Ia 85%, Ib-IIa 40%, IIb 25%, IIc-III 15%, IV <5%. The prognosis has changed very little in the last 30 years because women continue to present late in the disease process.

Effective screening would be of value if it were possible to detect disease in its early stages, thus enabling more effective treatment. Ultrasound scanning and various tumour markers (e.g. CA 125) are currently used.

Screening or prophylactic removal of the ovaries may be appropriate for women at increased risk of ovarian cancer as demonstrated by a strong and reliable family history (e.g. two or more first-degree relatives with ovarian cancer) or a mutation of the BRCA1 or BRCA2 gene.

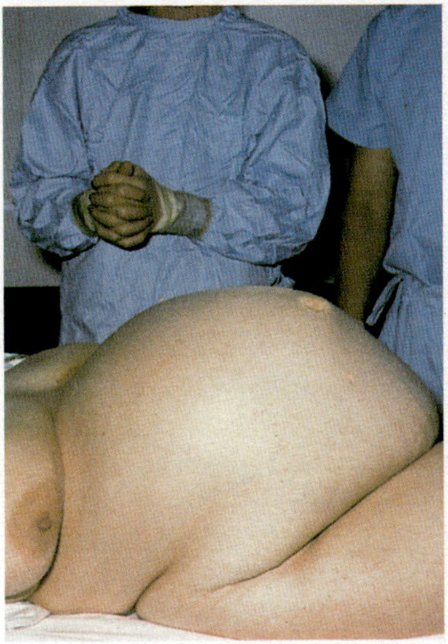

图 130　卵巢癌引起的巨大腹部膨隆
Gross abdominal distension due to ovarian tumour

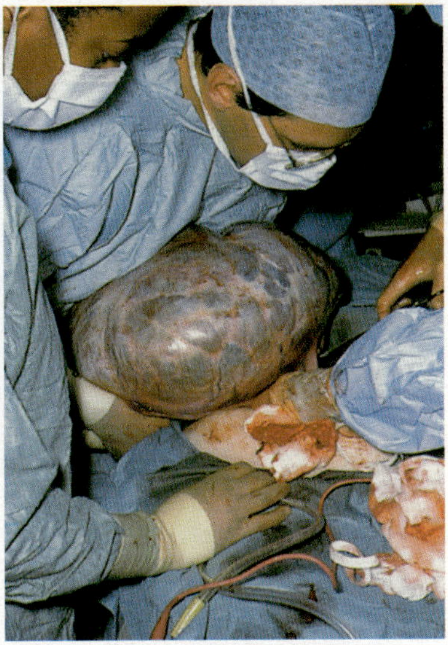

图 131　图 130 患者的开腹所见
Laparotomy findings in the case illustrated in Figure 130

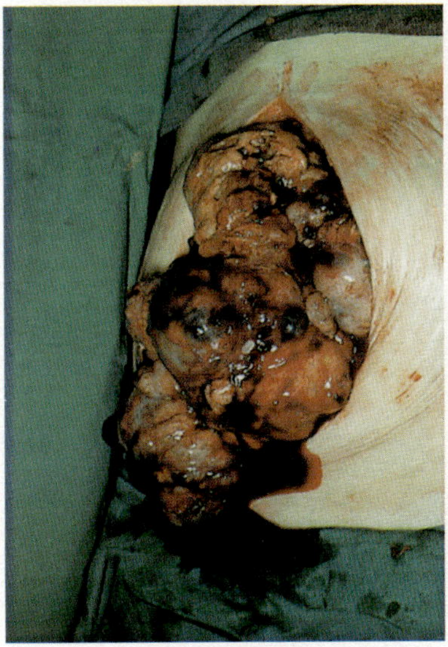

图 132　扩散的卵巢腺癌
Disseminated ovarian adenocarcinoma

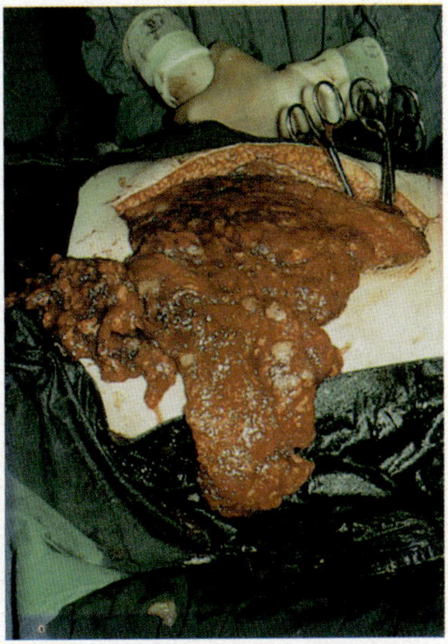

图 133　卵巢腺癌大网膜浸润
Omental infiltration with ovarian adenocarcinoma

绝经期和围绝经期

临床特征和病理学

定义

绝经期是女性最后的月经期；围绝经期是卵巢退化的时期，它包括绝经期。

病因

在围绝经期的初期，残存的卵巢内卵泡变得对促性腺激素的刺激越来越抵抗，因而促性腺激素产生增加以适应雌激素水平降低。

病理学

萎缩发生在所有对雌激素敏感的组织，如泌尿生殖系统、乳房和皮肤。骨骼也发生改变。骨质疏松定义为单位体积骨的骨组织数量减少，导致结构弱化。随着雌性激素的水平下降，成骨细胞功能降低和骨吸收能力增强。这造成了骨结构减弱和发生骨折的危险增加。最常见的骨折部位是桡骨、股骨颈和脊椎（图 134）。

由于绝经期的雌激素水平低下，心血管疾病发病率也随之上升。总胆固醇和低密度脂蛋白胆固醇水平升高，而高密度脂蛋白降低。这些脂质的改变可以解释增加的风险，其他的因素比如葡萄糖耐量改变和雌激素对动静脉血流的直接影响可能很重要。

骨质疏松被形容为“隐形流行病”，因为这种病很难被发现，直到女性摔倒，使骨质疏松的骨骼发生骨折。脊柱的楔状骨折可以通过 X 线发现（图 135）。如果是多处骨折，可能产生“贵妇人驼背”(dowager’s hump)。

The menopause and climacteric

Clinical features and pathology

Definition

The menopause is a woman's last menstrual period; the climacteric is the period of ovarian decline which includes the menopause.

Aetiology

At the beginning of the climacteric, the remaining ovarian follicles become increasingly resistant to gonadotrophin stimulation, and so more gonadotrophins are produced in response to the decreasing oestrogen levels.

Pathology

Atrophy occurs in all tissues that are sensitive to oestrogen, e.g. the urogenital system, breasts and skin.

Changes can also occur in bone. Osteoporosis is defined as a decreased amount of bony tissue per unit volume of bone, leading to structural weakness. With lowered oestrogen levels there appears to be a decrease in osteoblast function and an increase in bone resorption. This leads to a structural weakness in bone and increases the risk of fracture. The most common sites of fracture are the radius, the neck of the femur and the vertebral spine (Fig. 134).

Cardiovascular disease also increases with the lowered oestrogen levels of the menopause. An increase in total cholesterol and low-density lipoprotein cholesterol occurs, along with a decline in high-density lipoprotein. While these lipid changes account for increased risk, other factors such as changes in glucose tolerance and the direct effects of oestrogen on arterial and venous blood flow are likely to be important.

Osteoporosis is described as the 'silent epidemic' in that the disease may not be detected until the woman falls and fractures her osteoporotic bone(s). Wedge fractures of the spine may be detected on X-ray (Fig. 135) and, if multiple, may produce the 'dowager's hump'.

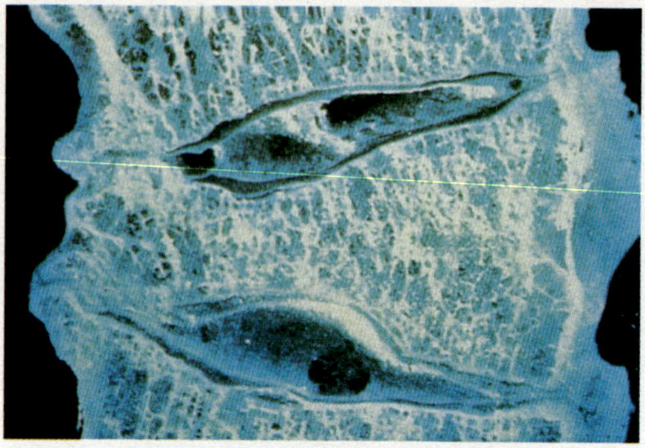

图 134　绝经后骨质疏松楔形骨折的标本
Post-mortem specimen of osteoporotic wedge fracture

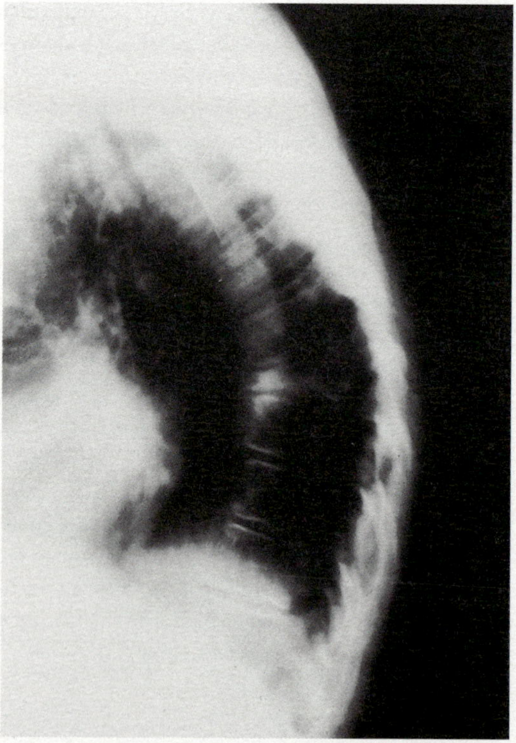

图 135　X 线显示胸椎楔形骨折
X-ray showing wedge fracture of thoracic spine

临床特征

潮热、盗汗是绝经期的典型症状。其他的症状包括情绪低落、阴道疼痛、阴道干涩、尿频、头痛和关节痛。在检查中还可能发现脱发、皮肤干燥和阴道萎缩。

检查

如果没有确诊，FSH 水平高于每升 15IU 将证实为卵巢衰竭。

现在有评价骨密度的非侵入性方法。起初使用单光子吸光分析，而后使用双光子吸光分析，现使用双能量X线作为放射线的来源（DXA，图136）。髋骨的骨吸光分析显示在图 137 上。

如有适应证应检查血压、乳房和宫颈细胞学。应该考虑乳房 X 线摄影。

治疗

激素替代治疗是对具有低雌激素症状的妇女和防治骨质疏松最适合的治疗。

给药有多种不同方法（图 138）。

口服　雌激素片剂是连续给药，孕激素片剂每月给予 12 日。对于绝经后女性（自末次月经已一年），雌激素和孕激素联合制剂连续应用可避免每月的流血。

肠道外途径　有经皮贴片或雌激素软膏。雌二醇植入片可每六个月进行皮下植入。性活跃妇女，可以同时植入睾酮植入片来促进性欲。当在阴道内使用软膏、阴道栓剂和环时可以提供局部治疗。

当有子宫时，以上所有制剂都必须同时给孕激素。

并发症

激素替代治疗与浸润性乳癌和静脉血栓栓塞性疾病发生风险增高有关。

Clinical features

Hot flushes and night sweats are the classic symptoms of the menopause. Other symptoms include depression, vaginal soreness, vaginal dryness, urinary frequency, headaches and joint pains. On examination, hair loss, dry skin and vaginal atrophy may be present.

Investigations

If the diagnosis is in doubt, an FSH level of greater than 15iu per litre will confirm ovarian failure.

Non-invasive methods are now available to assess bone density. Single photon absorptiometry was initially used, then dual photon, and now dual energy X-rays are used as the radioactive source (DXA, Fig. 136). Bone densitometry results of the hip are shown in Figure 137.

Blood pressure, breasts and cervical cytology should be checked as indicated. Mammography should be considered.

Management

Hormone replacement therapy is the most appropriate treatment for women with hypo-oestrogenic symptoms and for osteoporosis prevention.

There are various methods of administration (Fig. 138).

Oral Oestrogen tablets are given continuously and progestogen tablets are given for 12 days of each calendar month. For postmenopausal women (i.e. 1 year since LMP), continuous combined preparations of oestrogen and progestogen can be used to avoid monthly bleeding.

Parenteral Transdermal patches or oestrogen creams are available. Estradiol implants can be inserted subcutaneously every 6 months; a testosterone implant may be inserted at the same time if the woman is sexually active, to improve libido. Creams, pessaries or rings provide local treatment when used in the vagina.

With all the above preparations, progestogens must be given if there is a uterus.

Complications

HRT is associated with an increased risk of invasive breast carcinoma and venous thromboembolic disease.

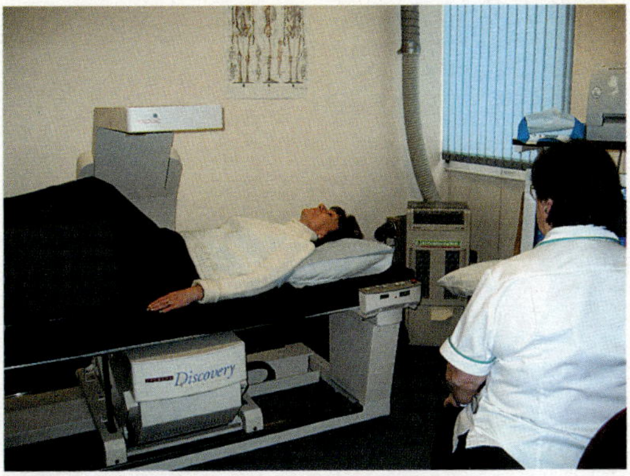

图 136　正在进行骨密度测量

Bone density measurement being performed

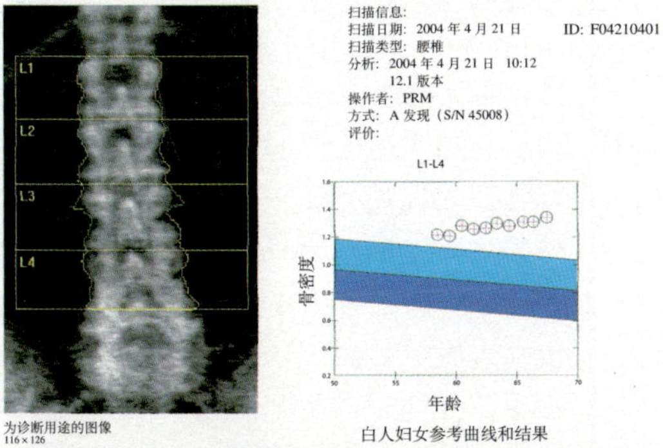

图 137　骨密度 DXA 输出

DXA printout of bone density

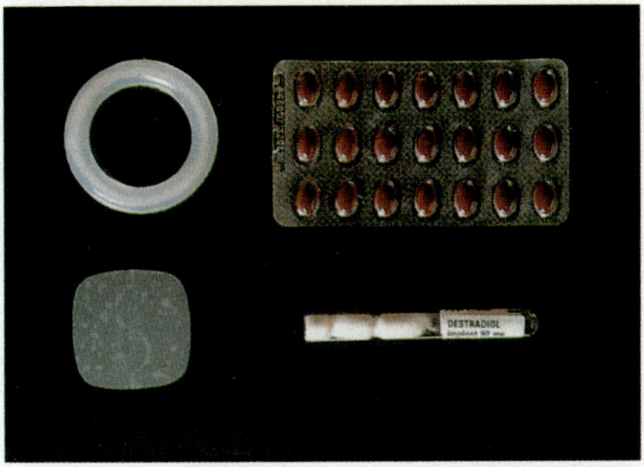

图 138　激素替代治疗——植入体、贴片、口服片剂、阴道环

HRT — implant, patch, oral tablets, vaginal ring

18 子宫阴道脱垂

定义

阴道前壁由耻骨宫颈韧带支持。这条韧带从耻骨联合后面伸展到宫颈和阴道上部。阴道后壁由直肠阴道隔的纤维组织和肛提肌支持。子宫主要是由主韧带或宫颈横韧带支持，上述韧带在进入宫颈前与宫骶韧带合并。

子宫阴道脱垂是子宫位置下降（图139），和/或阴道下降或超出阴道口。膀胱、尿道、直肠和肠管也可能受影响。

阴道壁膨出

阴道前壁下1/3膨出包括尿道，称为尿道膨出。阴道前壁上2/3处膨出包括膀胱，称为膀胱膨出（图140）。当阴道后壁的下部脱垂时也使直肠下降，因此称之为直肠膨出。在此以上的阴道壁膨出，包括直肠子宫陷凹，被称作肠疝（图141）。

病因

在未生育过的女性中不常见，如出现是由于骨盆支撑结构先天较薄弱。绝大部分有脱垂的女性都生过孩子。分娩时骨盆韧带组织和盆底肌肉的神经供应受损，导致后来的薄弱。其他因素促成或加剧上述结果，包括绝经后骨盆支撑组织的萎缩和腹部压力的慢性增加，如伴有肥胖或慢性咳嗽。

Uterovaginal prolapse

Definition

The anterior vaginal wall is supported by the pubocervical fascia. This extends from the back of the symphysis pubis to the cervix and upper vagina. The posterior vaginal wall is supported by fibrous tissue of the rectovaginal septum and the levator ani muscles. The uterus is supported mainly by the cardinal or transverse cervical ligaments, which merge with the uterosacral ligaments before joining the cervix.

Uterovaginal prolapse is the downward displacement of the uterus (Fig. 139) and/or vagina towards or through the introitus. The bladder, urethra, rectum and bowel may also be involved.

Vaginal wall prolapse

A prolapse of the lowest one-third of the anterior vagina involves the urethra and is called a urethrocele. Prolapse of the upper two-thirds of the anterior vaginal wall involves the bladder and is therefore called a cystocele (Fig. 140). When the lower portion of the posterior vaginal wall prolapses, it brings with it the rectum and is therefore termed a rectocele. Prolapse of the vaginal wall above this involves the pouch of Douglas; it is called an enterocele (Fig. 141).

Aetiology

Uncommon in nulliparous women, where it is due to congenital weakness of the pelvic supporting structures. The majority of women with prolapse have had children. Childbirth is associated with damage to the ligamentous tissues of the pelvis and nerve supply of the pelvic floor muscles, causing later weakness. Other factors contributing to or exacerbating these effects include postmenopausal atrophy of pelvic-supporting tissue and chronic raised intra-abdominal pressure, e.g. with obesity or chronic cough.

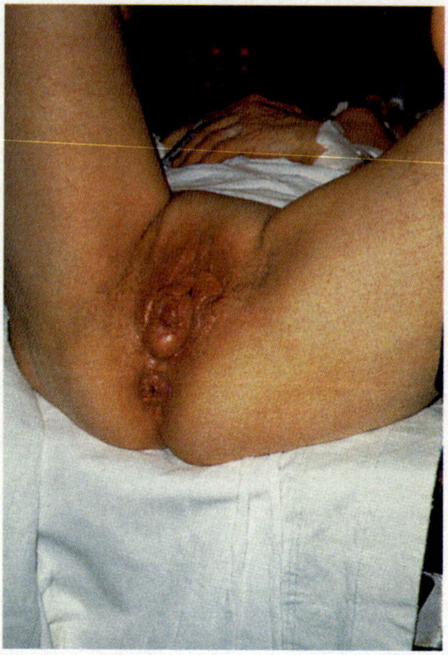

图 139　脱垂
Procidentia

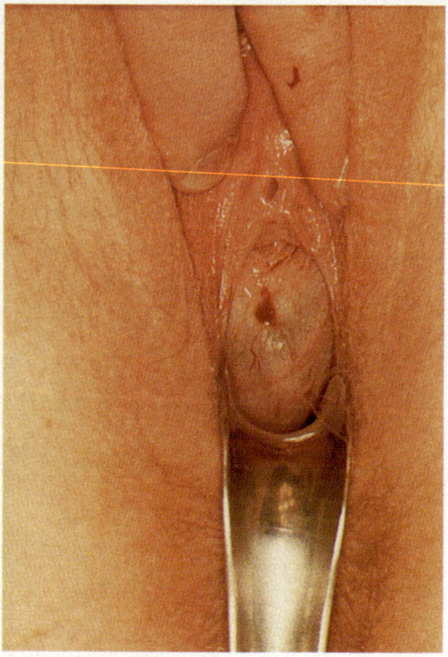

图 140　膀胱膨出
Cystocele

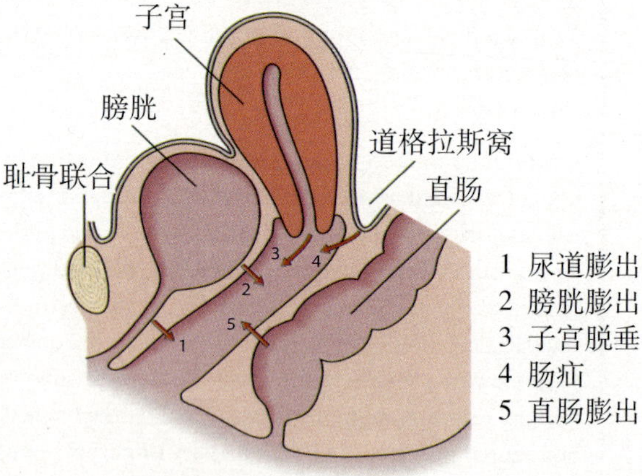

图 141　阴道膨出
Prolapse of the vagina

临床特征

病人可能描述有种“下坠”感，并且有块状物自阴道口脱出。尿失禁与尿道膨出有关。膀胱突出严重时可出现尿潴留。排便困难也可能出现。疼痛不是脱垂的特征，但可能出现日益严重的下坠不适感和后背疼。

处理

预防 避免损伤性的阴道分娩，提倡产前和产后的骨盆底锻炼。对已过绝经期的女性，倡导不吸烟和适当的使用激素替代疗法。

保守疗法 当女性不适合或不想接受外科手术及在两次怀孕中间，环型和架型宫托（图 142）是适合的短期疗法。

手术治疗 方法包括:

- *阴道前壁修补术*: 适用于膀胱膨出患者，但对于张力性尿失禁患者不是最适合的疗法。
- *阴道后壁修补术*: 适用于直肠膨出患者。
- *阴式子宫切除术*: 是对子宫脱垂患者的一种疗法，必要时常同前后壁修补术同时使用（图 143）。
- *曼彻斯特修补术（Fothergill 修补术）*: 包括缩短宫颈横韧带并切除宫颈，同时行前壁修补术。对于子宫体支撑良好而宫颈延长、凸出的患者，它是很有效的手术。

发生在子宫切除术后的阴道穹窿膨出可以通过经腹或腹腔镜下骶棘韧带固定术或通过将阴道固定于骶椎而纠正。

并发症

长期使用子宫托会造成阴道溃疡。阴道手术的短期并发症有出血、血肿形成、感染和尿潴留。切口裂开和肠管自阴道膨出（图 144）非常罕见。长期来看，阴道狭窄和性交痛可能发生。脱垂也可能复发。

Clinical features

Patients may describe a feeling of something 'coming down', and there is the presence of a lump protruding through the vulva. Urinary incontinence may be associated with a urethrocele. Urinary retention may be seen when a large cystocele is present. Difficulty with defaecation may also be present. Pain is not a feature of prolapse but dragging discomfort and backache that worsen throughout the day may be experienced.

Management

Prophylaxis Avoid traumatic vaginal deliveries and encourage antenatal and postnatal pelvic floor exercises. Discourage cigarette smoking and use hormone replacement therapy appropriately in postmenopausal women.

Conservative treatment Rings and shelf pessaries (Fig. 142) are a suitable short-term option in women unfit or not keen to undergo surgery, and between pregnancies.

Surgery Procedures include:

- *Anterior repair*: corrects a cystocele but may not be the most appropriate treatment for stress incontinence
- *Posterior repair*: corrects a rectocele
- *Vaginal hysterectomy*: is the treatment of choice in uterine prolapse and is combined with anterior and posterior repairs as necessary (Fig. 143)
- *Manchester (Fothergill) repair*: involves shortening the transverse cervical ligaments and amputating the cervix, together with an anterior repair. It is a useful operation when the uterine body is well supported, but the cervix is elongated and protruding

A vaginal vault prolapse occurring after hysterectomy can be corrected by a sacrospinous fixation or by securing the vagina to the sacrum abdominally or laparoscopically.

Complications

Long-term use of pessaries can cause vaginal ulceration. Immediate complications of vaginal surgery include haemorrhage, haematoma formation, infection and urinary retention. Wound breakdown and extrusion of bowel through the vagina (Fig. 144) are extremely rare. In the longer term, stenosis and dyspareunia may result. Prolapse may also recur.

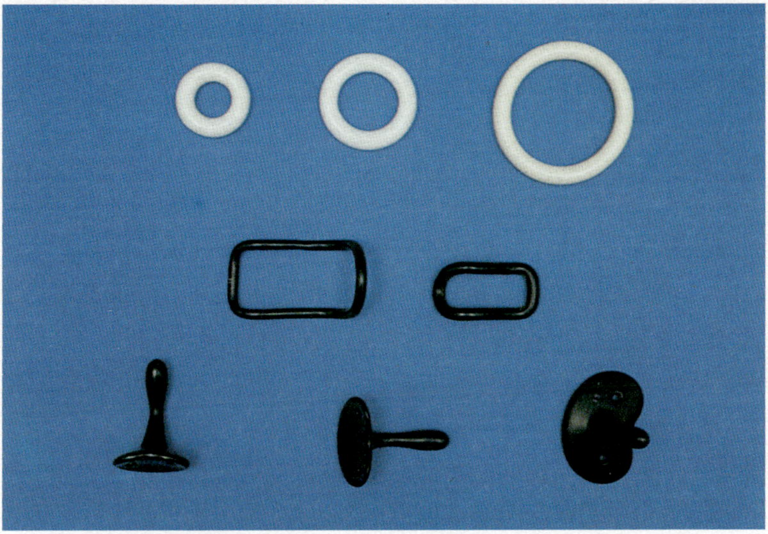

图 142　环型和架型子宫托，用于减轻膨出
Rings and shelf pessaries used to relieve prolapse

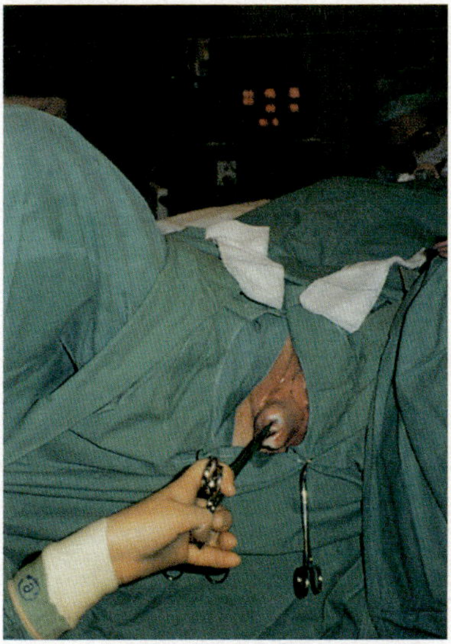

图 143　阴式子宫切除术开始时的脱垂
Procidentia at commencement of vaginal hysterectomy

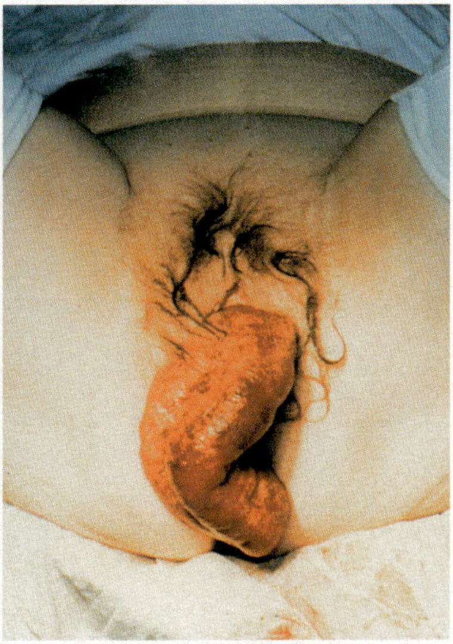

图 144　肠疝——阴式子宫切除术罕见的并发症
Bowel herniation —a rare complication of vaginal hysterectomy

急迫性尿失禁

定义 由不能抑制的逼尿肌收缩引起的尿液不自主溢出。

病因 绝大多数病例为特发性的，逼尿肌不自主收缩引起尿急、尿频，当膀胱内压力超过尿道内压力时，就引起尿失禁。

临床特征 病史会有尿频、尿急、夜尿，也可能有尿失禁，检查通常无异常。

检查 收集中段尿标本进行显微镜检查和培养，如有任何迹象提示“混合”现象，如急迫症状和压迫症状，尿动力学检查（图 145）是必要的。称重法可以用来评估尿失禁。也可应用膀胱尿道 X 线造影术。

处理 *膀胱肌锻炼*　需要患者的推动和意识上的生物反馈。嘱患者每隔一定时间排尿一次，然后间隔时间逐渐增加，直至达到间隔 3 或 4 小时。

药物治疗　钙通道阻滞剂、抗胆碱药、神经节阻滞剂、雌激素替代和节后神经节阻滞。

手术治疗　Clam膀胱成形术、膀胱横切和骶神经切除术很少使用，仅用于疑难病例。

并发症 症状复发很常见。膀胱扩张可能会导致膀胱破裂。术后可能会有膀胱排空困难。

Urge incontinence

Definition Involuntary loss of urine caused by uninhibited detrusor contractions.

Aetiology Most cases are idiopathic. The detrusor contracts in an uninhibited fashion, causing urgency and frequency, and when the intravesical pressure exceeds the intraurethral pressure, incontinence results.

Clinical features The history will reveal urinary frequency, urgency, nocturia and, perhaps, incontinence. On examination there is usually no abnormality.

Investigations A mid-stream urine specimen should be taken for microscopy and culture. If there is any suggestion of a 'mixed' picture, i.e. symptoms of urge as well as stress, urodynamic investigations are essential (Fig. 145). Padweighing can be used to assess incontinence. Videocystourethrography is also useful (Fig. 146).

Management *Bladder drill* This requires patient motivation and ideally biofeedback. The patient is told to pass urine at certain time intervals, which are then gradually increased until 3 or 4 h is reached.

Drug therapy Calcium antagonists, anticholinergic agents, ganglion blockers, oestrogen replacement and postganglion blockers.

Surgery Clam cystoplasty, bladder transection and sacral neurectomy are rarely used and are reserved for difficult cases.

Complications Recurrence of symptoms is common. Bladder rupture can occur with cystodistension. Voiding difficulties can occur after surgery.

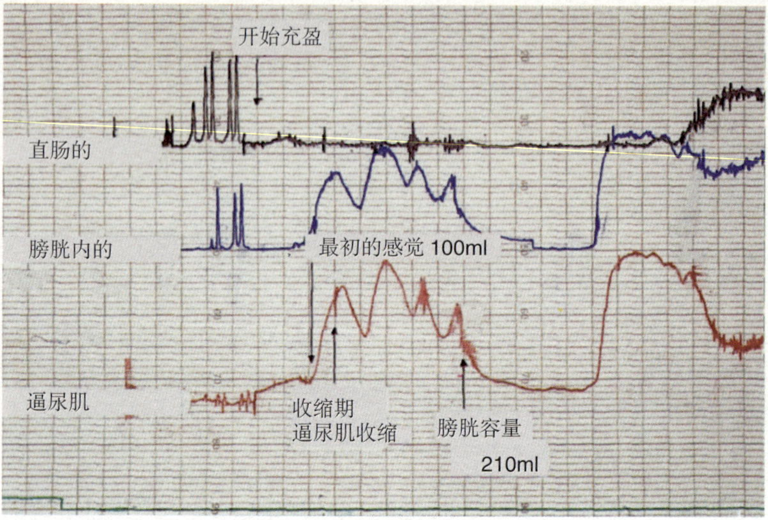

图 145　膀胱内压测量法显示稳定的膀胱
Cystometry readout showing a stable bladder

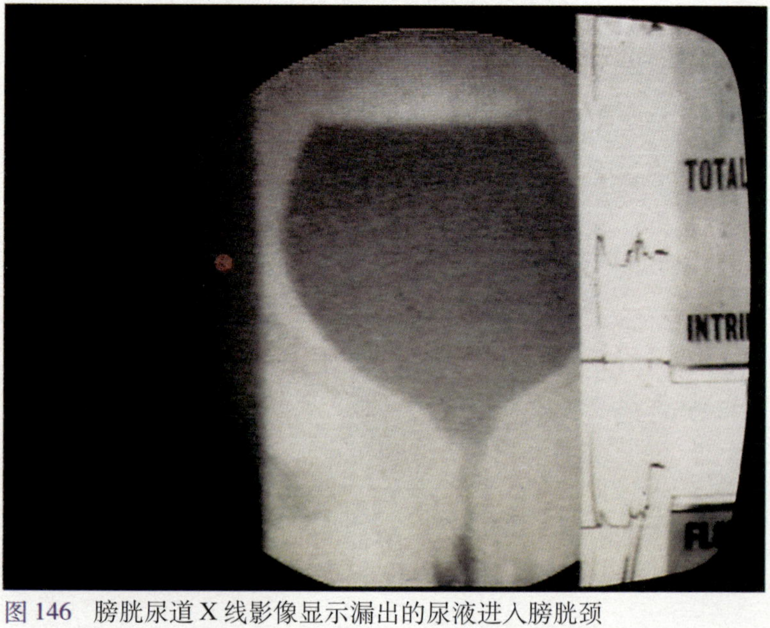

图 146　膀胱尿道 X 线影像显示漏出的尿液进入膀胱颈
Leakage of urine into bladder neck seen on videocystourethrography

真性压力性尿失禁

定义 腹压升高时发生的尿液不自主溢出。

病因 为先天性的或继发于多产、阴道脱垂、绝经或手术前的尿道括约肌松弛。

临床特征 大笑、咳嗽或打喷嚏时尿液不自主流出。查体可见外阴由于持续潮湿而造成的脱皮。患者可采用西姆斯体位，插入西姆斯窥器以显示阴道前壁，嘱患者咳嗽（假如膀胱不空虚）可以见到尿液溢出。可能有膀胱膨出。

处理 首先应治疗感染。其他治疗方法包括：

- *物理治疗*：盆底肌肉锻炼加阴道锥（图 147）或感应电疗法可有效。
- *阴道悬吊术*：通过尿道和膀胱颈旁缝合使膀胱颈提高，通过开腹或腹腔镜手术可以完成。
- *无张力阴道吊带术（tension-free vaginal tape, TVT）步骤*：将一个编织的Prolene网带置于尿道中段，悬吊至前腹壁；目的是使吊带在无压力时自由放置，在咳嗽时给予阴道足够的压力，阻止尿液溢出（图 148）。
- *膀胱前壁修补术*：切开阴道前壁，使尿道提高。
- *注射药物*：把 GAX 胶原或大塑料溶胶注射至尿道旁，使括约肌周围膨胀。
- *吊带*：使用有机材料或无机材料。
- *内镜下膀胱颈悬吊*：适用于复发性压力性尿失禁患者
- *人造括约肌*

并发症 膀胱排空困难是术后常见症状，压力性尿失禁的复发并非罕见。如有原发性逼尿肌不稳定，那么手术效果不佳。

预后 膀胱悬吊术的治愈率为90%，膀胱前壁修补术治愈率为 40% ~ 60%。

Genuine stress incontinence

Definition

Involuntary loss of urine when intra-abdominal pressure rises.

Aetiology

Urethral sphincter weakness, which is either congenital or secondary to multiparity, prolapse, menopause or previous surgery.

Clinical features

The patient gives a history of losing urine involuntarily when she laughs, coughs or sneezes. On examination the vulva may be excoriated due to persistent wetness. If the patient is placed in the Sims position and a Sims speculum is inserted to display the anterior vaginal wall, urine loss may be demonstrated when the patient is asked to cough (providing her bladder is not empty). A cystocele may be present.

Management

Infection should be treated. Other treatments include:

- *Physiotherapy*: involving pelvic floor exercises with cones (Fig.147) or faradism can be effective
- *Colposuspension*: the bladder neck is elevated by inserting sutures beside the urethra and bladder neck. This can be done using an abdominal incision or laparoscopically
- *Tension-free vaginal tape (TVT) procedure*: a knitted Prolene mesh tape is placed mid-urethra and is brought up through the anterior abdominal wall; the aim is to have the tape lying free at rest and only exerting sufficient pressure on the urethra during a cough to prevent leakage of urine (Fig.148)
- *Anterior colporrhaphy*: the urethra is elevated from below after opening up the anterior vaginal wall
- *Injectables*: GAX collagen or macroplastique is injected paraurethrally to build up bulk around the sphincter
- *Slings*: organic or inorganic material is used.
- *Endoscopic bladder neck suspensions*: are useful for recurrent stress incontinence
- *Artificial sphincters*

Complications

Following surgery, voiding difficulties are common and recurrence of the stress incontinence is not uncommon. The results of surgery are poor if detrusor instability was present originally.

Prognosis

Colposuspensions have a 90% cure rate and anterior colporrhaphies 40%~60%.

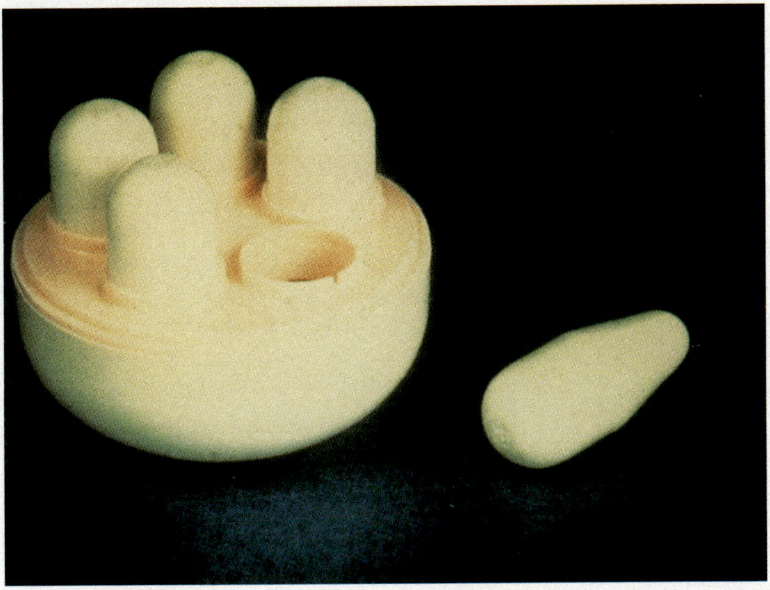

图 147 阴道锥
Vaginal cones

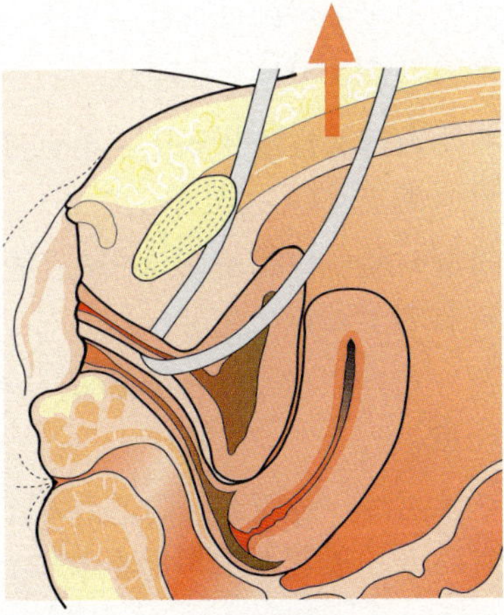

图 148 无张力阴道吊带
Tension-free vaginal tape

溢流性尿失禁

定义 少量尿液频繁且不自主地溢出、尿流缓慢以及尿不净感。

病因 由于膀胱弛缓，而使膀胱流出受阻，原因有：自主神经损害、药物、手术、盆腔肿物、子宫阴道脱垂、局部炎症或固化。

临床特征 询问病史可发现以上症状。检查可见增大的膀胱，插入导尿管后可引出大量残余尿。

检查 中段尿（mid-stream urine，MSU）

膀胱内压测量法 出现第一感觉延迟，膀胱容积增大。最大排空压力正常或增加，峰值流出率变缓。排尿时膀胱尿道造影（图 149）。尿流流量仪。

治疗 根据病因选择治疗。神经性疾病是不能治愈的，可以学习间歇性自行导尿术。

真性尿失禁

定义 持续性尿失禁。

病因 通常继发于梗阻性分娩、手术、肿瘤或放疗形成的瘘管（图 150）。

临床表现 有阴道持续性溢尿病史。检查可见瘘管，尿液染色可有助于定位。

检查 排尿时膀胱尿道造影术和/或静脉肾盂造影术检查可有助于定位。

处理 *保守治疗* 取决于病因，有一些患者可以随时间痊愈。

手术治疗 经腹或经阴道手术。如果有组织糟碎，可以去除瘘管，用植皮术治疗。

并发症 压力性尿失禁、阴道瘢痕、复发。

Overflow incontinence

Definition
Frequent involuntary loss of small volumes of urine, slow urinary stream and a postmicturition feeling of incomplete emptying.

Aetiology
Obstruction to bladder outflow in bladder atony which can be due to motor neurone lesions, drugs, surgery, pelvic mass, uterovaginal prolapse, local inflammation or immobilization.

Clinical features
History will reveal the above symptoms. Examination will demonstrate an enlarged bladder, and catheterization will produce a large residual volume of urine.

Investigations
MSU (mid-stream urine)

Cystometry will demonstrate a delayed first sensation and a large bladder capacity. Maximum voiding pressure will be normal or increased, and the peak flow rate will be slow. Micturating cystourethrogram (Fig. 149). Uroflowmeter.

Treatment
This will depend on the cause. Neurological causes are not treatable and intermittent self-catheterization can be learned.

True incontinence

Definition
Continuous incontinence.

Aetiology
Usually due to a fistulous track (Fig. 150) secondary to obstructed labour, surgery, carcinoma or radiotherapy.

Clinical features
There will be a history of continuous draining of urine from vagina. Examination may reveal the track, and colouring the urine may aid location.

Investigations
A micturating cystourethrogram and/or an IVP may help location.

Management
Conservative. Depending on aetiology, some may heal with time.

Surgery can be performed abdominally or vaginally. The fistulous track is removed and an interposition graft used if the tissues are poor.

Complications
Stress incontinence, vaginal scarring and recurrence.

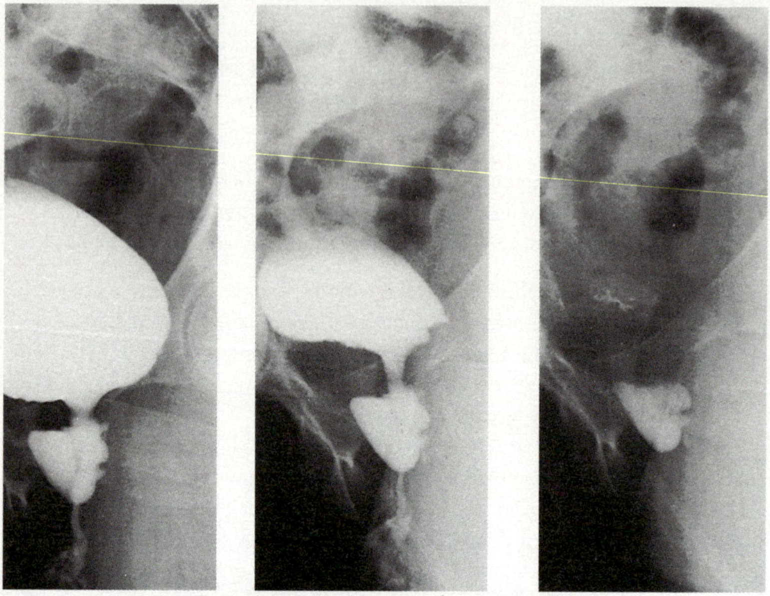

图 149　排尿时膀胱造影术显示大的尿道憩室
Micturating cystogram demonstrating large urethral diverticulum

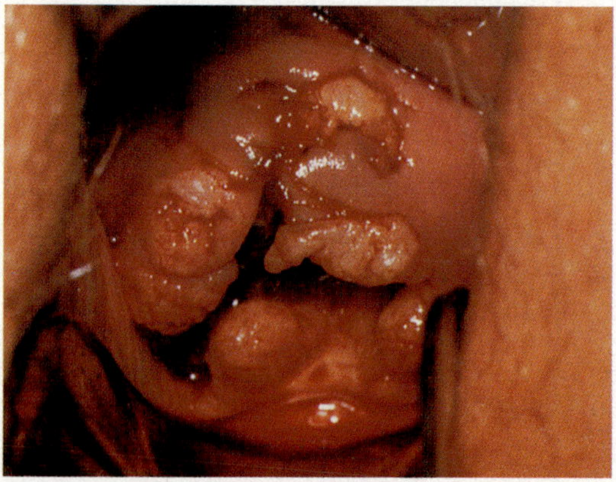

图 150　通过阴道黏膜不规则碎片可见膀胱黏膜
Bladder mucosa visible through irregular fragments of vaginal mucosa

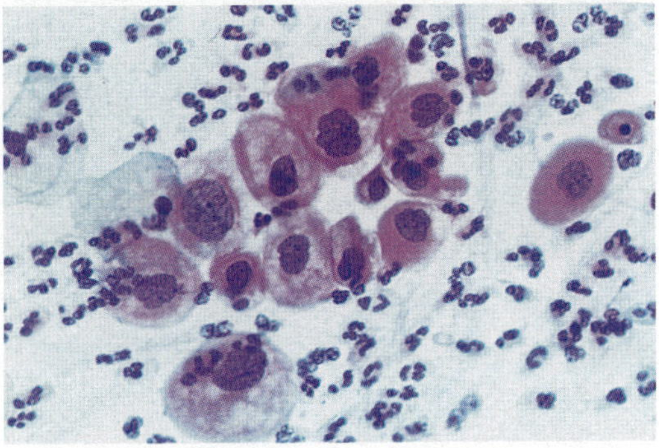

1. 该载玻片显示的是染色体核型异常。

a. 显示的是何种细胞？

b. 这些细胞显示某些恶性特征，请说出它们。

c. 如何处理？

This slide shows dyskaryosis.

a. What type of cells are these?

b. These cells display some of the features of malignancy. Name them.

c. What is the management?

2. a. 该检查使用的是何种窥器？

b. 描述放置该窥器的体位。

c. 何种情况下使用该窥器？

d. 使用该窥器时还需配合使用何种器具？

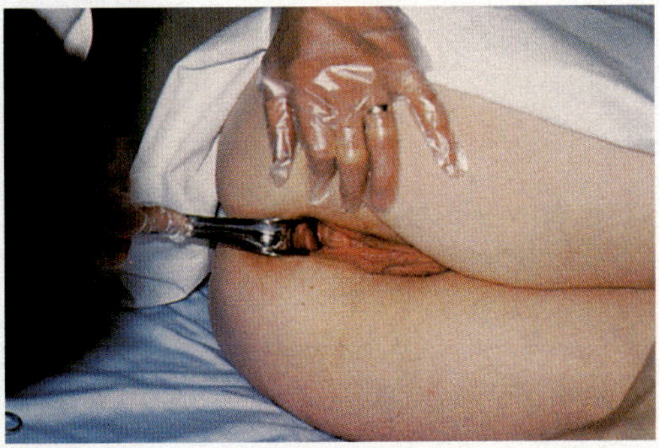

a. What speculum is being used for this examination?

b. Describe the Sims position.

c. In what circumstances would you use this speculum?

d. What other instruments should you use with this speculum?

3. a. 这些是什么？
b. 它们的作用机制是什么？
c. 绝对禁忌证是什么？
d. 试述如何放置？
e. 使用它们的并发症是什么？
f. 含铜节育器需多久更换一次？

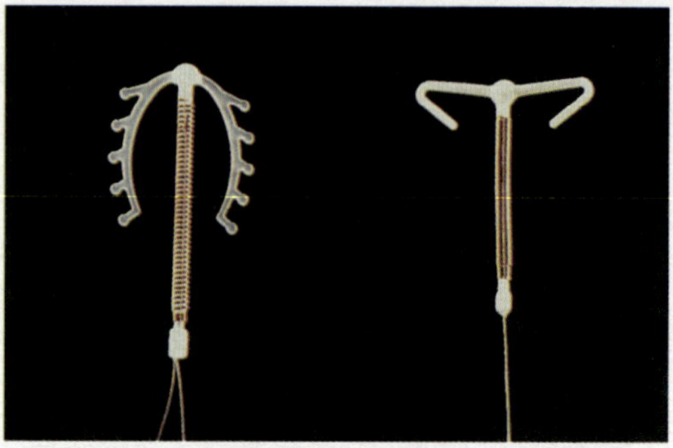

a. What are these?
b. What is the mechanism of action?
c. What are the absolute contraindications?
d. Describe the mechanism of insertion.
e. What are the complications associated with their use?
f. How often should copper-containing devices be changed?

4. a. 诊断为何病？
b. 患者主诉为什么？
c. 如何确诊？
d. 如何处置？
e. 如何处理病情较顽固者？

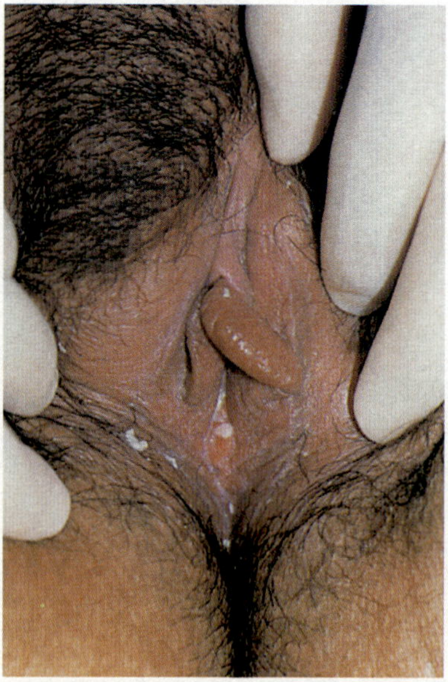

a. What is the diagnosis?
b. What symptoms may the patient complain of?
c. How would you confirm the diagnosis?
d. What is the treatment?
e. How would you treat the recalcitrant case?

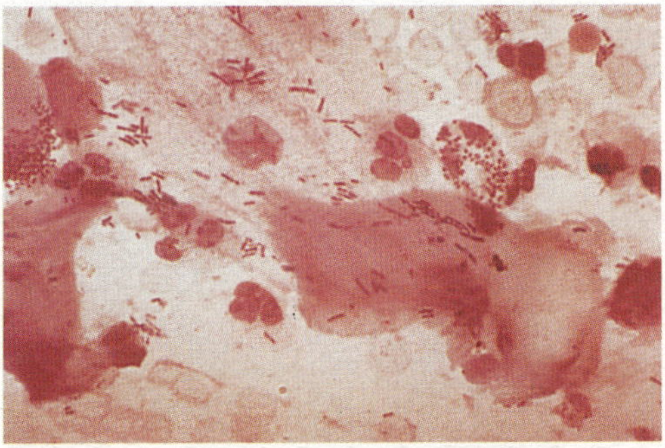

5. a. 这张革兰染色涂片显示的是何种病原体?
b. 可导致何种临床情况?
c. 女性患者的临床表现是什么?
d. 如何确诊?
e. 治疗原则是什么?

a. What organisms are present on this Gram-stain smear?
b. What is the resultant clinical condition?
c. What are the clinical manifestations in females?
d. How is the definitive diagnosis made?
e. What are the principles of management?

6. a. 该女孩所患何病?
b. 此类患者有何临床表现?
c. 分娩过程中会出现什么情况?
d. 可采用何种妇科治疗来减轻这一症状?
e. 如果在分娩过程中诊断，如何助娩?

a. What procedure has this young girl undergone?
b. How may these patients present?
c. What problems can occur in labour?
d. What elective gynaecological procedure can alleviate the problem?
e. If diagnosed in labour how may delivery be facilitated?

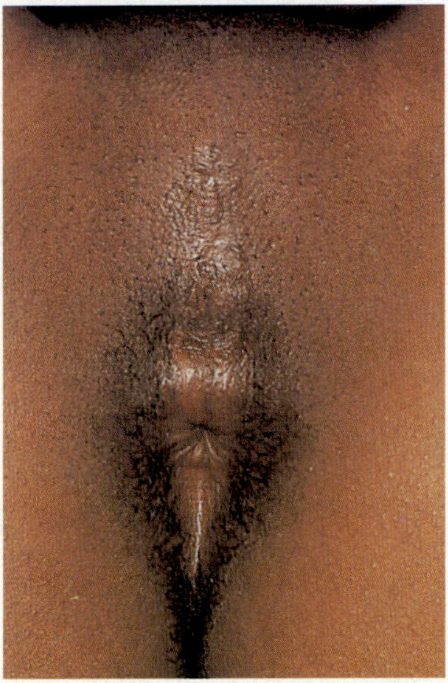

7. a. 该X线片提示何种情况？
b. 还可用何种影像学技术来确诊？
c. 最可能的病因是什么？患者通常因何就诊于妇科？
d. 你还将对病人进行何种检查？
e. 说出高泌乳素血症的其他病因。
f. 如何治疗？

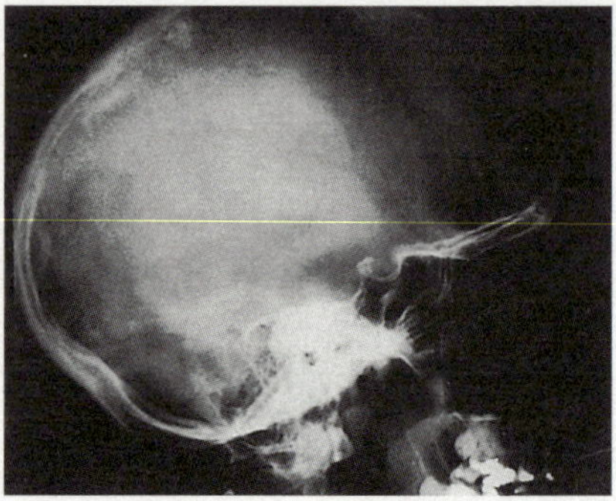

a. What does this X-ray reveal?
b. What other imaging techniques can be used to make the diagnosis?
c. What is the most likely cause and how would this patient present to the Gynaecology Department?
d. What other investigations would you perform?
e. Name other causes of hyperprolactinaemia.
f. What are the treatment options?

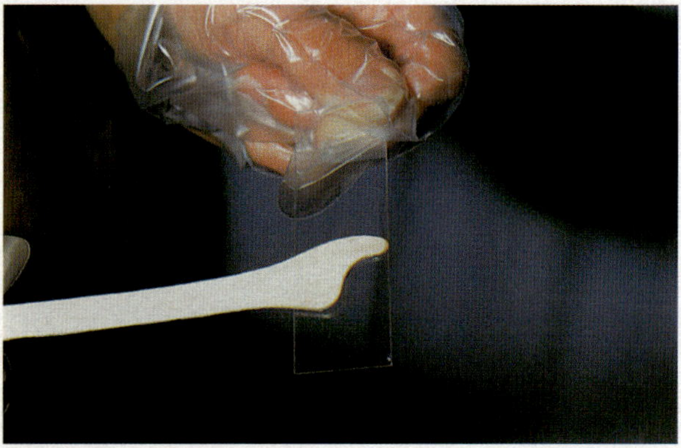

8. a. 现正进行何种检查？检查的目的是什么？
b. 该器具的名称是什么？
c. 应多久进行一次该检查？
d. 在何部位取样？
e. 如何获得最佳的取样？

a. What test is being performed and what is the purpose?
b. What is the name of the instrument?
c. How frequently should this investigation be performed?
d. What area must be sampled?
e. How can one optimize the sample obtained?

9. a. 明显的诊断是什么?
b. 何年龄组易发生该病?
c. 何种组织类型最常见?
d. 主要的转移途径是什么?
e. 治疗原则是什么?

a. What is the obvious diagnosis?
b. In what age group does this condition typically occur?
c. What is the usual histology?
d. What is the primary route of spread?
e. What are the principles of treatment?

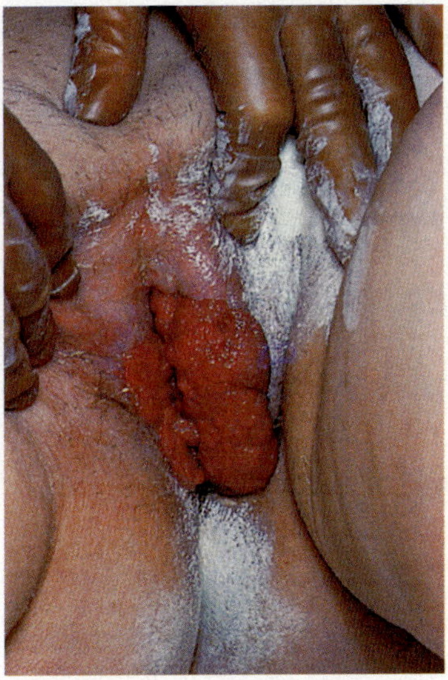

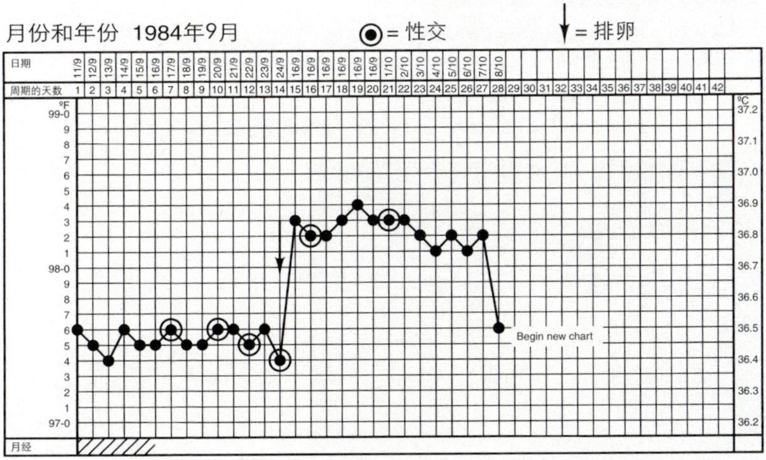

10. a. 这是什么图表?
b. 该图表说明什么问题?
c. 通过该图表可推测出什么变化?
d. 通过何种方法可确诊该变化?

a. What is the name of this record?
b. What does this record illustrate?
c. What event has presumptively occurred?
d. By what method can this event be more definitively diagnosed?

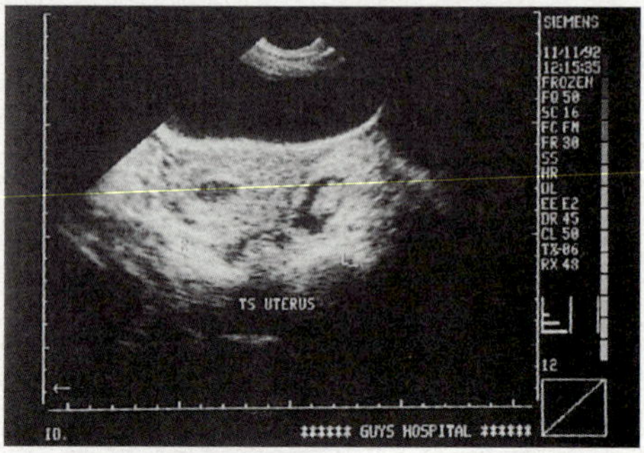

11. 该图为未破裂型宫外孕患者的超声图。

a. 描述超声学改变。

b. 此病变的典型症状是什么？

c. 典型的体征是什么？

d. 何种辅助检查有助于诊断该病？

The photographs in questions 11-13 relate to a woman who presented with an unruptured ectopic pregnancy.

a. Describe the sonographic findings.

b. What are the classic symptoms of this condition?

c. What are the typical signs?

d. What ancillary investigations can help to make the diagnosis?

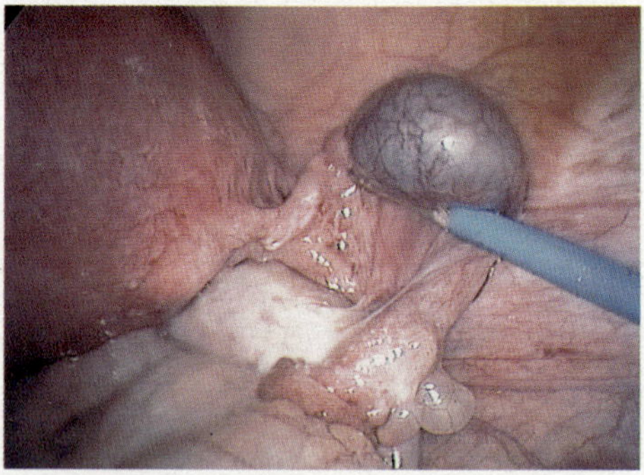

12. a. 导致异位妊娠发病的病因有哪些？

b. 通常发生于何解剖学部位？

c. 异位妊娠的自然病史是什么？

d. 鉴别诊断是什么？

a. What aetiological factors contribute to the incidence of ectopic pregnancy?

b. What are the common anatomical sites?

c. What is the natural history of ectopic pregnancy?

d. What is the differential diagnosis?

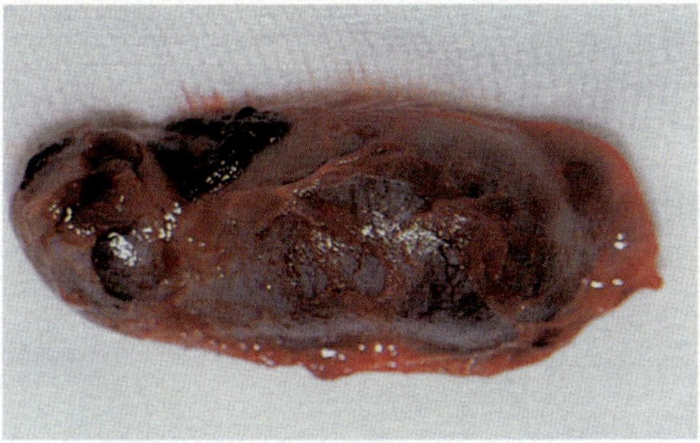

13. 该患者行输卵管切除术。
a. 治疗异位妊娠时有哪些方法?
b. 术后给予患者何种建议?
c. 再发风险多大?

This patient underwent salpingectomy.
a. What treatment options are available in the treatment of ectopic pregnancies?
b. How would you counsel this patient postoperatively?
c. What is the recurrence risk?

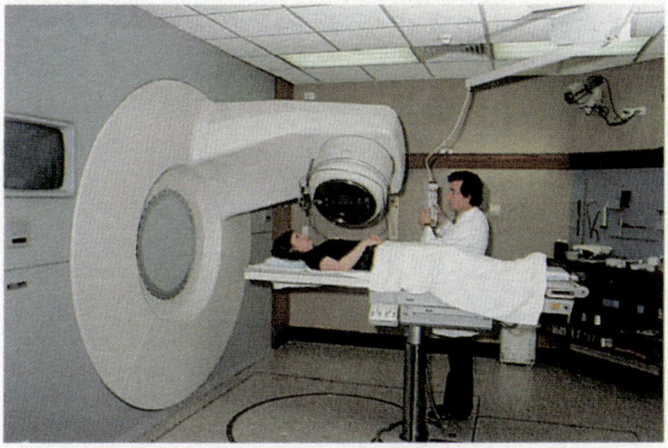

14. 该年轻妇女正接受放射治疗。
a. 放疗对哪些妇科癌症有确定的治疗作用?
b. 放疗的方式有几种?
c. 急性副反应有哪些?
d. 对盆腔器官的远期并发症有哪些?

This young woman is undergoing radiation therapy.
a. For which gynaecological cancers does radiation therapy have an established curative role?
b. In what ways may radiation therapy be delivered?
c. What acute adverse reactions are seen?
d. What are the possible long-term sequelae of radiation therapy to the pelvic region?

15. a. 最可能的诊断是什么？定义该疾病。
b. 该疾病的病因有哪些理论？
c. 该病症状和体征有哪些？
d. 此病例如何确诊？

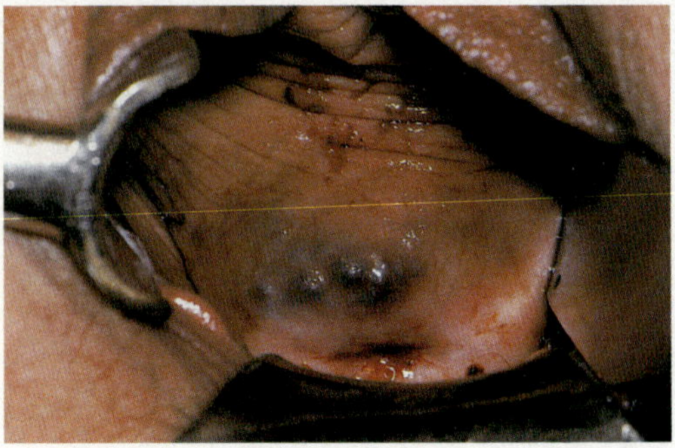

a. What is the most likely diagnosis? Define this condition.
b. What are the theories of aetiology?
c. What are the symptoms and signs?
d. How could the diagnosis be confirmed in this case?

16. a. 描述图中所见。
b. 诊断为何？
c. 该病变的基础是什么？
d. 此类患者何时出现症状？
e. 临床检查还可发现何改变？

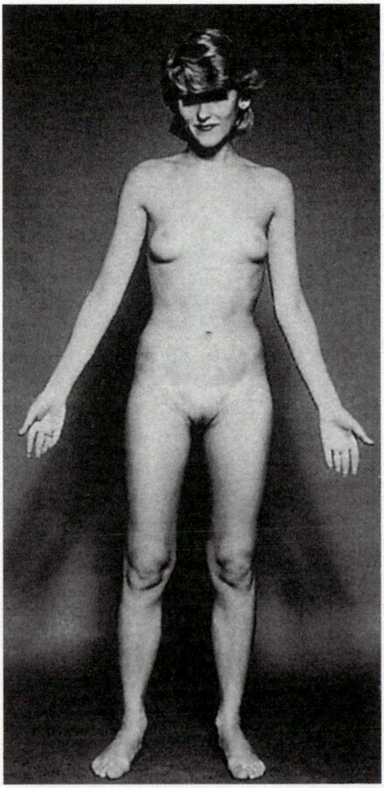

a. Describe what you see.
b. What is the diagnosis?
c. What is the basis of this condition?
d. When do these patients normally present?
e. What else might you find on clinical examination?

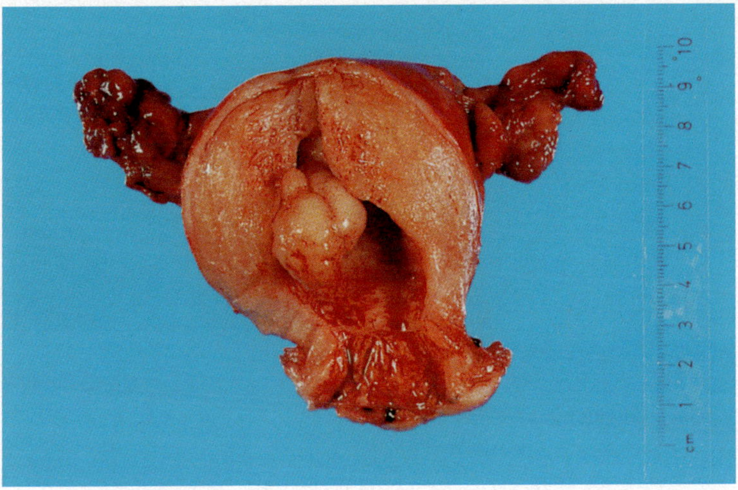

17. a. 描述图中所见。
b. 可能引起何种症状?
c. 如何检测此病变?
d. 如何治疗?

a. Describe what you see.
b. What symptoms may these cause?
c. How may these be detected?
d. What is the treatment?

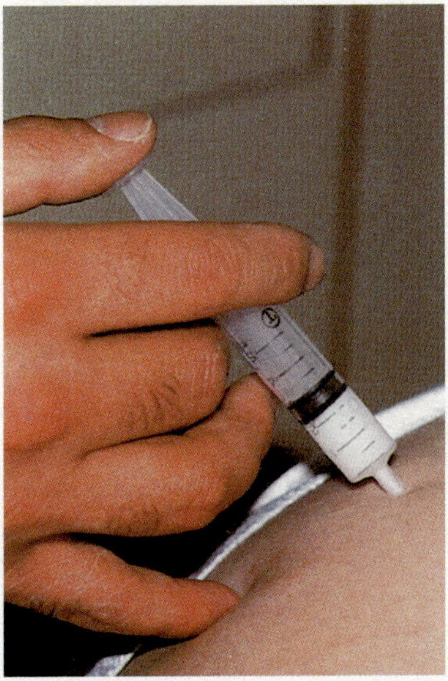

18. 该妇女正在被注射醋酸亮丙瑞林。
a. 该药的作用机制是什么?
b. 给予的剂量是固定的吗?
c. 此法的失败率是多少?
d. 此法的优点是什么?
e. 此法的缺点是什么?

This woman is receiving depot medroxy progesterone acetate.
a. How does it work?
b. Is a steady dose provided?
c. What is the failure rate of this method?
d. What are the advantages of this method?
e. What are the disadvantages?

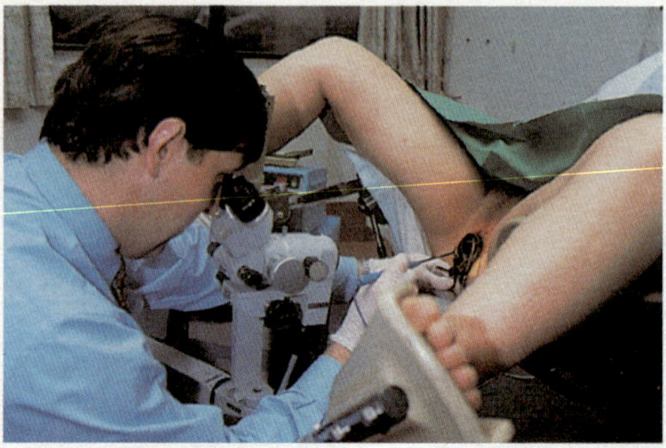

19. a. 此妇女正进行何种检查？
b. 哪些患者可进行此检查？
c. 此过程包括哪几个基本步骤？
d. 进行检查前，你对患者有何建议？

a. What investigation is this woman undergoing?
b. Who would you refer for this investigation?
c. What basic steps are involved in this procedure?
d. How would you counsel a woman prior to referral?

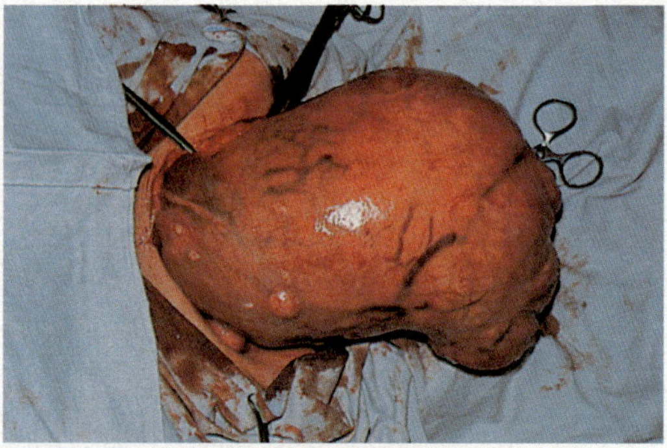

20. 这是一个患缺铁性贫血妇女的术中标本。
a. 什么原因导致贫血？
b. 患者术前可能有何种症状？
c. 术前应用何种药物可使手术易于操作？

This is an intraoperative specimen of a woman who had iron-deficiency anaemia.
a. What might have caused this anaemia?
b. What symptoms might she have presented with?
c. What preoperative medication can be prescribed to simplify surgery?

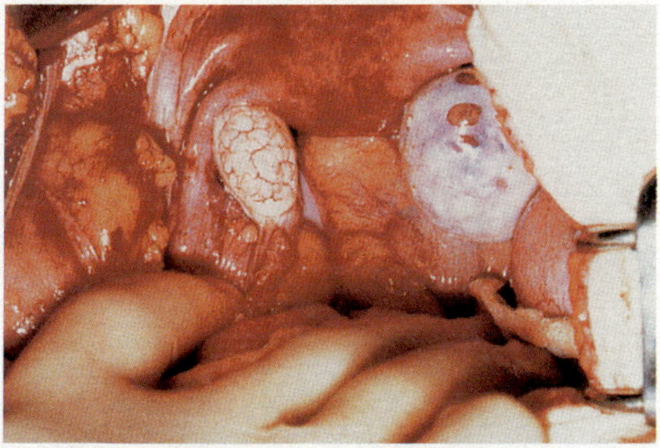

21．a. 列出对表现出男性化的患者的诊断进程。

b. 导致该患者男性化的病因是什么？

c. 何种卵巢肿瘤可产生雄激素并导致男性化？

d. 切除肿瘤后，哪些男性化的症状可消失？

a. Outline the diagnostic approach in a patient who exhibits virilism.

b. What cause of virilism is present in this patient?

c. Which ovarian tumours produce androgens and virilizing syndromes?

d. Which signs of virilism disappear after removal of such tumours?

22．a. 诊断为何？

b. 典型的临床表现是什么？

c. 应如何处理这种情况？

d. 该病的产科并发症是什么？

a. What is the diagnosis?

b. What are the typical clinical features?

c. How should this condition be managed?

d. What are the obstetric implications of this condition?

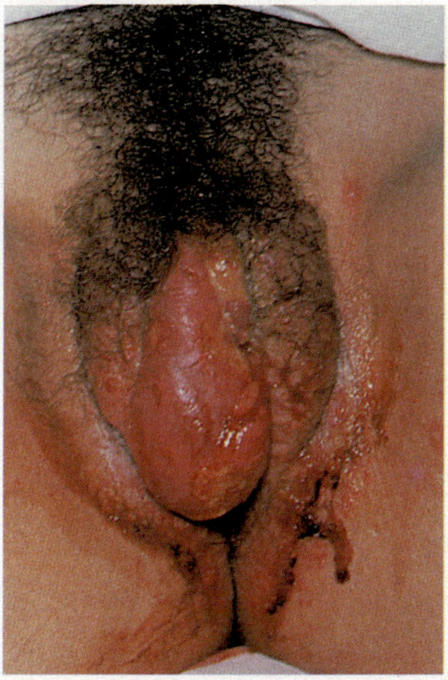

23. a. 诊断为何？
b. 此病的年龄分布如何？
c. 特征性的临床表现是什么？
d. 特征性的播散类型是什么？
e. 此病如何分期？
f. 详细说明这 4 个分期？

a. What is the diagnosis?
b. What is the age distribution of this condition?
c. What is the typical presentation?
d. What is the characteristic pattern of spread?
e. How is this condition staged?
f. Define the four stages.

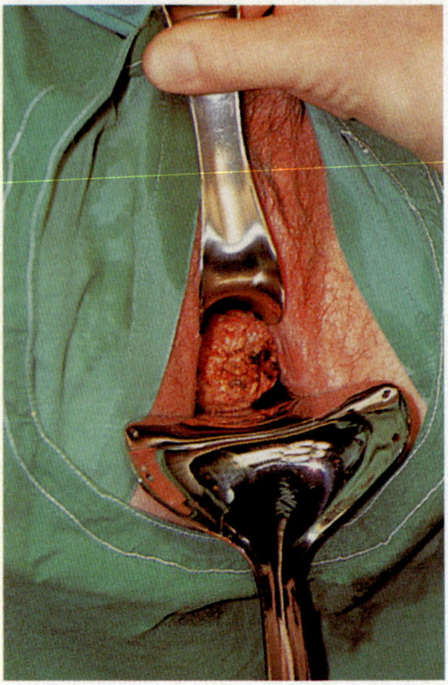

24. a. 这是什么窥器？
b. 患者采用的是何体位？
c. 如何放置窥器？
d. 还应进行何种检查以辅助该窥器的使用？

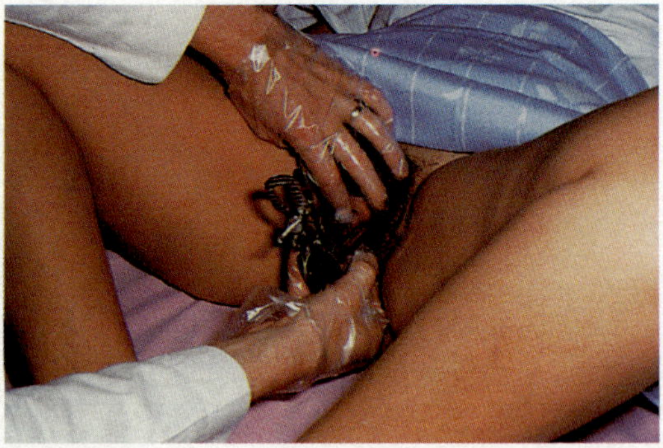

a. What is this speculum called?
b. What position is the patient in?
c. How would you insert this speculum?
d. What examination would you use as an adjunct to the use of this speculum?

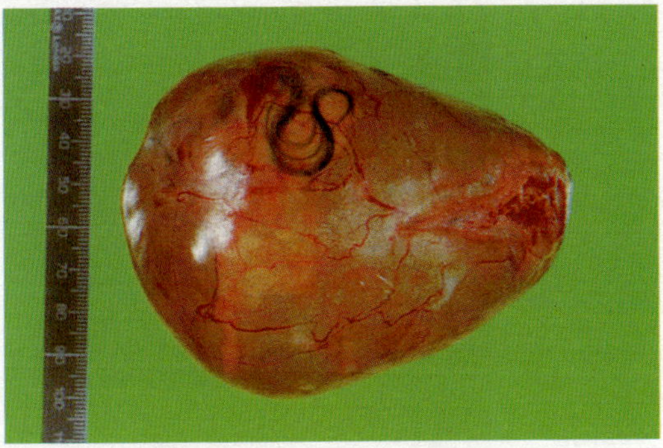

25. a. 诊断是什么?
b. 多见于哪一年龄组?
c. 囊肿起源于哪里? 囊肿内可包含哪些组织?
d. 双侧发病的几率有多大? 这一数据有何意义?
e. 恶性倾向有多大?

a. What is the diagnosis?
b. At what ages is this typically seen?
c. What is the origin of the cyst? What tissues can be within it?
d. What is the incidence of bilateral lesions and what is the significance of this figure?
e. What is the malignant potential?

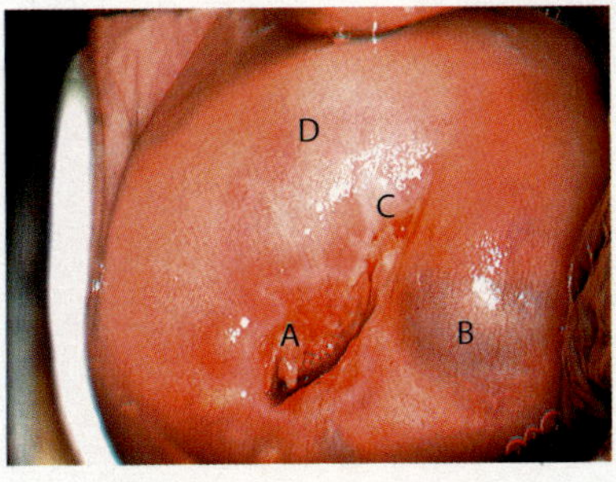

(a)

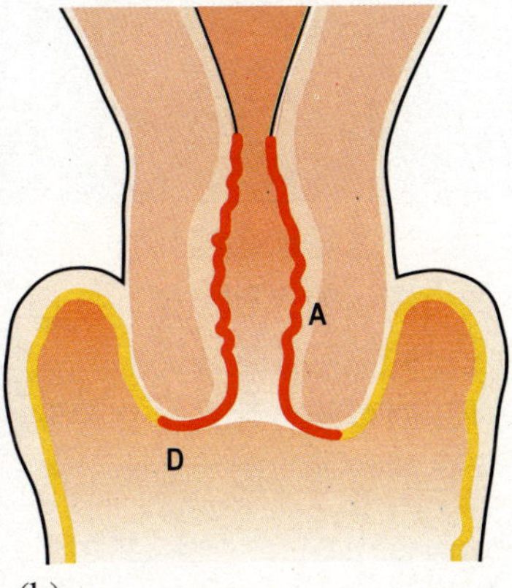

(b)

26. 辨别宫颈上标记的四个区。

Identify the four areas labelled on the cervix.

27. a. 此为何病？
b. 哪一评分体系可用来评价该病的严重程度？
c. 该病的常见病因是什么？
d. 你对患者做何检查？
e. 有哪些治疗方案？

a. What is the name of this condition?
b. What scoring system can help estimate the severity of the problem?
c. What are the common causes?
d. How would you investigate this patient?
e. What treatment modalities are available?

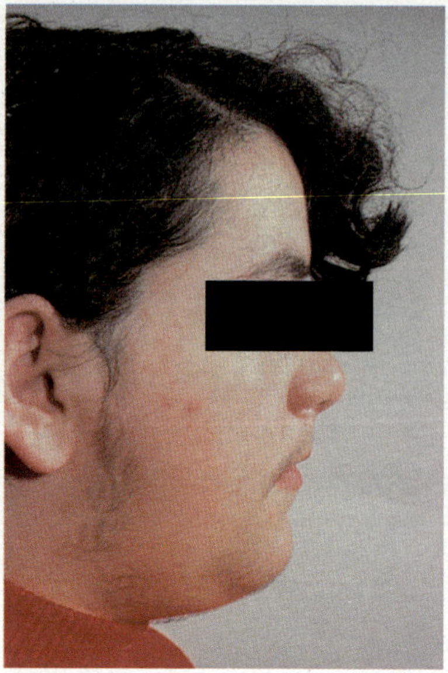

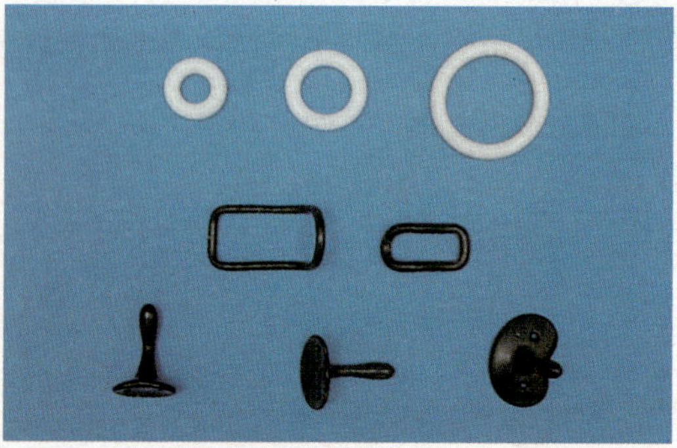

28. a. 这些是什么器具？
b. 说出图示的三种类型。
c. 使用的适应证是什么？
d. 使用时可能有哪些潜在并发症？
e. 白色的器具应多久更换一次？

a. What are these devices called?
b. Name the three types illustrated.
c. What are the indications for their use?
d. What potential complications can occur with their use?
e. How often should the white devices be changed?

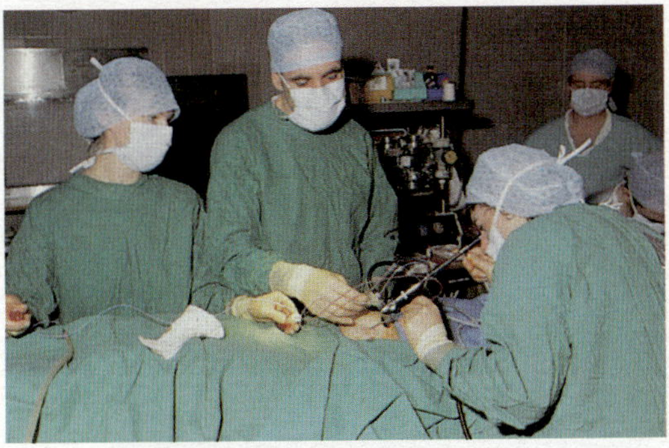

29. a. 正在进行何种操作？
b. 向腹腔内充盈的是什么？
c. 此方法可看到何器官？
d. 在 Veress 针刺入前，应让病人做什么？

a. What procedure is being performed?
b. What is the peritoneal cavity inflated with?
c. What organs can be visualized by this method?
d. What must be done before the Veress needle is introduced?

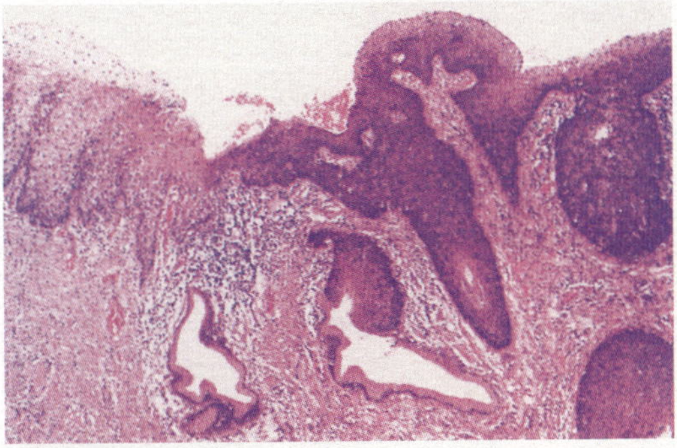

30. 这是一张宫颈切片。
a. 图中显示何病变？
b. 有浸润的迹象吗？
c. 如果经锥切病变被完全切除，如何安排随访？
d. 预计该患者治疗前的涂片显示什么？

This is a slide of a cervix.
a. What does it show?
b. Is there evidence of invasion?
c. If the lesion was completely excised by cone biopsy, what follow-up would you arrange?
d. Prior to treatment what would you anticipate the smear on this woman to reveal?

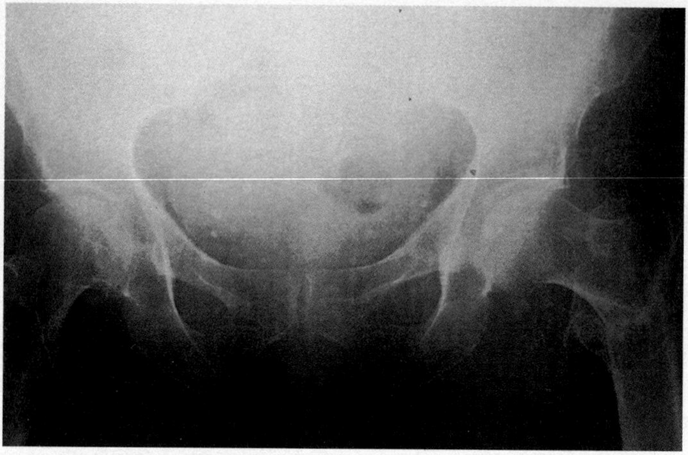

31. a. 此图显示为何？
b. 说出可能的潜在病变。
c. 还有哪些部位受该病变影响？
d. 病因是什么？
e. 对妇女健康的长期影响是什么？

a. What does this photograph show?
b. Name the probable underlying pathology.
c. What other sites are affected by the underlying pathology?
d. What are the causes of the underlying problem?
e. What are the long-term implications for this woman's health?

32. a. 该图示的两个诊断是什么？
b. 通常症状是什么？
c. 这一潜在疾病的危险因素是什么？
d. 脊柱中何种类型的骨占优势？
e. 图示疾病可引起的何种生活方式的改变？

a. What are the two diagnoses present?
b. What are the usual symptoms?
c. What are the risk factors for the underlying disease?
d. What type of bone predominates in the spine?
e. What are the lifestyle implications for the conditions illustrated?

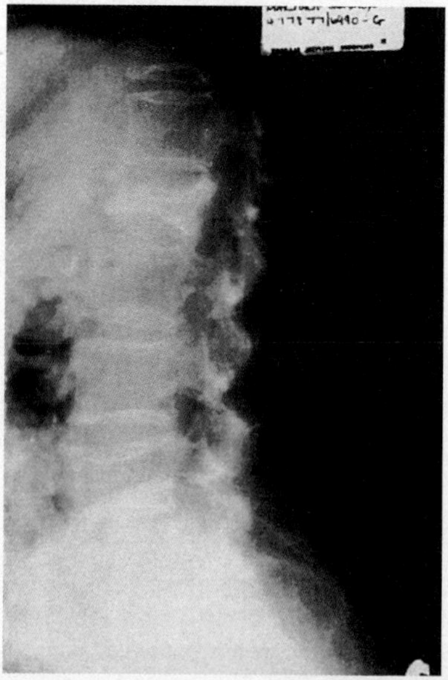

33. a. 图示为何种检查？
b. 在什么年龄妇女骨量达到峰值？
c. 何种方法有助于增加骨量峰值？
d. 与年龄相关的骨质丢失是什么？
e. 绝经期妇女骨量丢失的速率是多大？

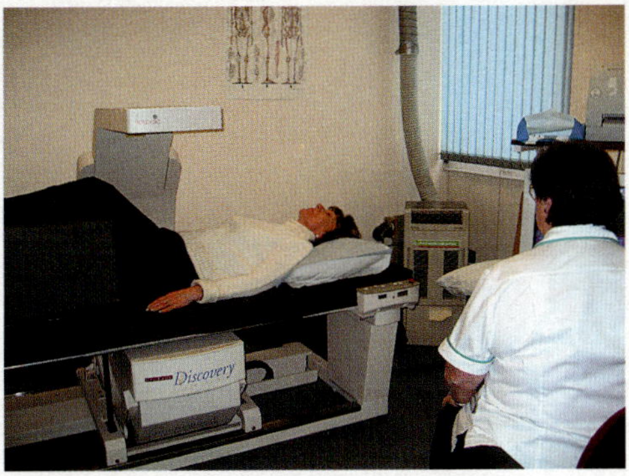

a. What is this examination?
b. At what age does a woman attain peak bone mass?
c. What measures can help to maximize the peak bone mass?
d. What is the age-related rate of bone loss?
e. What is the rate of bone loss following the menopause?

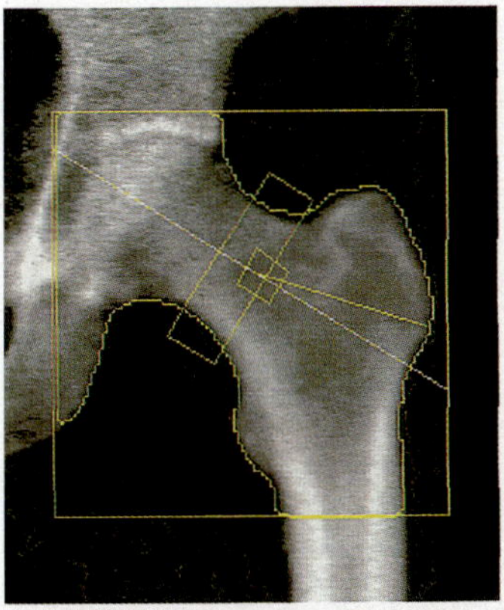

Image not for diagnostic use
101 x 103

扫描信息：
扫描日期：2004 年 4 月 21 日　　ID: F0421040K
扫描类型：左臀
分析：2004 年 4 月 21 日　10:16　版本　12.1
　　　左臀
操作者：PRM

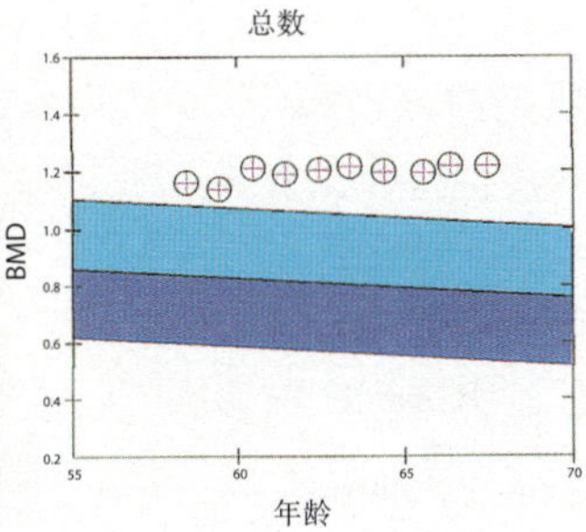

34. a. 该图是如何产生的？
b. 正在测量的是什么？
c. 还可采用何种其他方法测量？
d. 什么是 Ward 三角？
e. 与其他方法相比，此法有何优点？

a. How was this image produced?
b. What is being measured?
c. What other tests are available to obtain this measurement?
d. What is Ward's triangle?
e. What are the advantages of this test over the other methods?

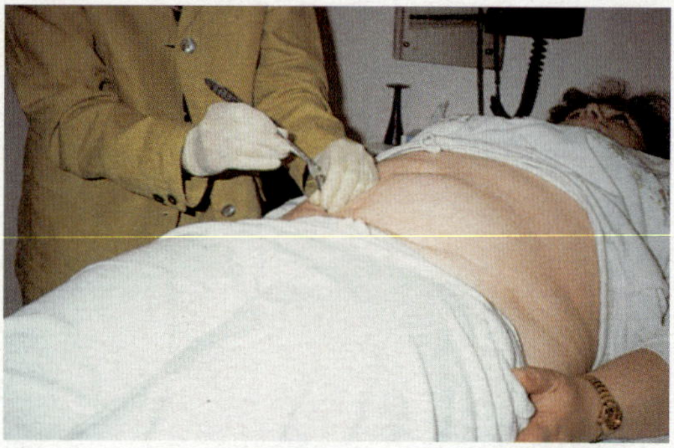

35. a. 正进行的是何种操作?
b. 成分是什么?
c. 为何要给予这种治疗?
d. 多久给药一次?
e. 需要加用孕激素吗?

a. What is the procedure that is being performed?
b. What is the likely ingredient?
c. Why are these administered?
d. How often are they administered?
e. Should progestogens be given as well?

36. a. 这是何种疾病?
b. 染色体核型是什么?
c. 典型体征是什么?
d. 该患者有可能自然妊娠吗?
e. 如何对该病进行产前诊断?

a. What is this condition?
b. What is the characteristic karyotype?
c. What are the typical physical findings?
d. Is spontaneous pregnancy a possibility for this person?
e. How can this condition be diagnosed antenatally?

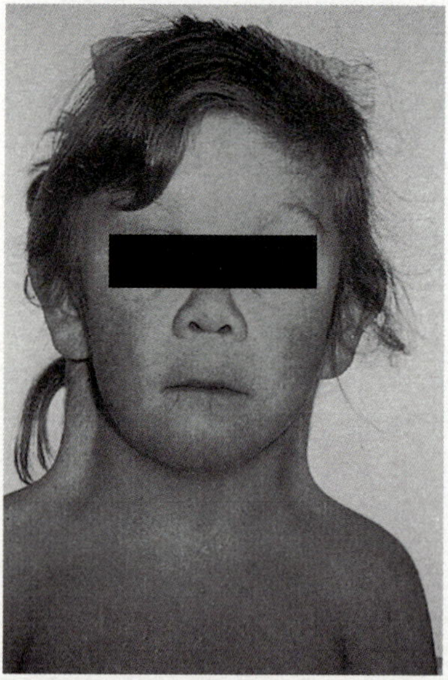

37. 这是刮宫获得的组织物。

a. 图示的是什么?

b. 诊断为何?

c. 典型症状是什么?

d. 体征是什么?

e. 如何治疗?

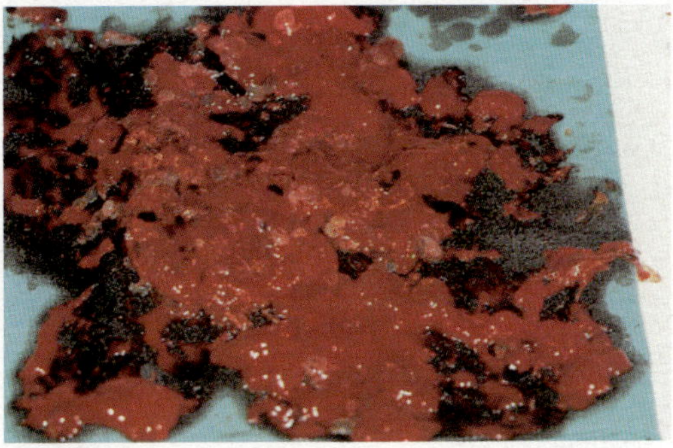

This tissue was removed at a D&C.

a. What does this illustrate?

b. What is the diagnosis?

c. What are the typical symptoms?

d. What are the signs?

e. What is the management?

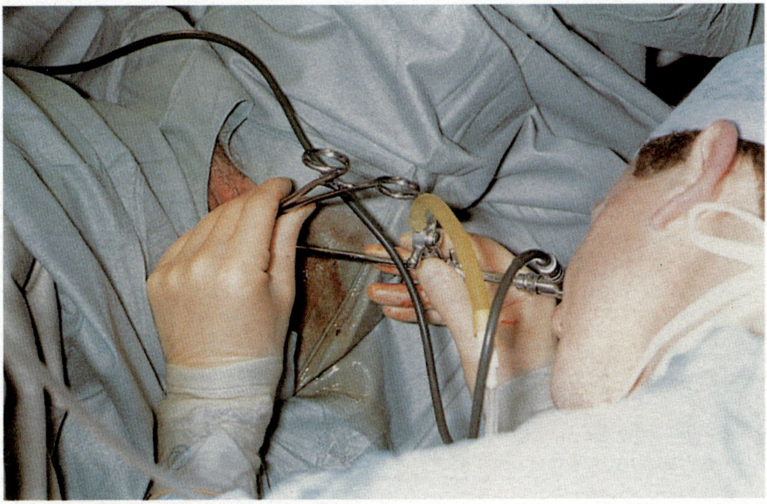

38. 该妇女表现为绝经后流血。

a. 正进行何种检查?

b. 橡胶管中输入的是什么物质?

c. 该检查有何作用?

This woman presented with postmenopausal bleeding.

a. What investigation is being performed?

b. What is being passed through the rubber tubing?

c. What does this operation enable you to do?

39. a. 这是什么检查方法？
b. 描述图中所见。
c. 该患者会有何泌尿系症状？
d. 有哪些妇科疾病会导致如图所示的改变？

a. What investigation has been performed?
b. Describe the findings.
c. With what urinary symptoms may this patient present?
d. What gynaecological causes may result in this picture?

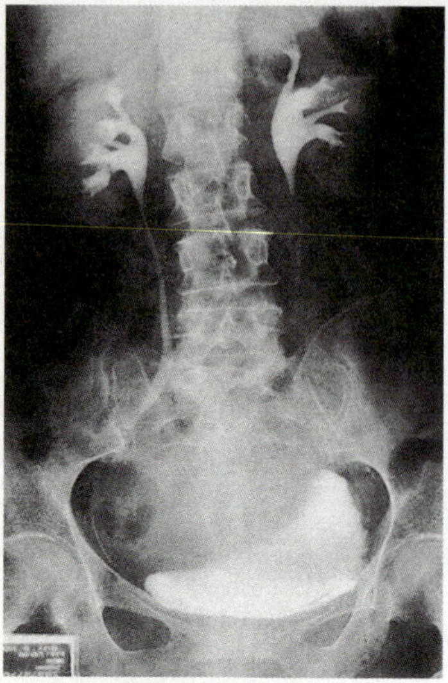

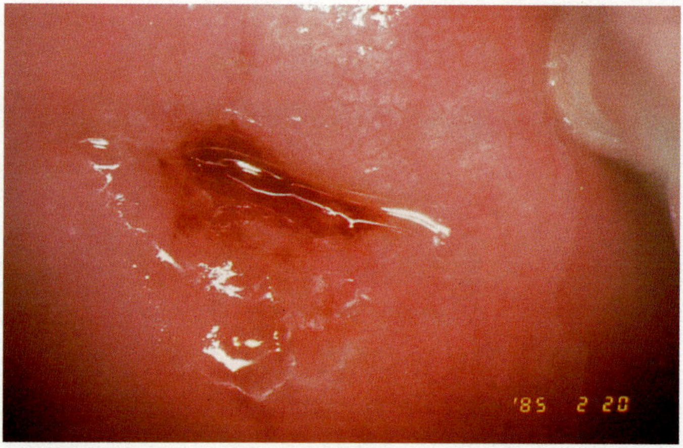

40. a. 用于宫颈上的是何种溶液？
b. 能观察到什么？
c. 你认为这是一个严重的病变还是轻微病变？
d. 活检显示这是 CIN Ⅰ。请描述 CIN Ⅰ。
e. 它能自发消退吗？

a. What solution has been used on the cervix?
b. What can you see?
c. Do you think this is a severe or a minor lesion?
d. A biopsy showed CIN I. Describe CIN I.
e. Can spontaneous regression occur?

精液分析报告	
我们实验室的正常数据在括号中给出：它们是建立在射精1小时内并且禁欲3～5天的样品之上。	
临床数据：低生育能力调查	
患者出生日期：24/12/69	
产生的时间：10:10 hr	**到达实验室时间**：10:15hr
禁欲：6 天	**体积**：2.5ml (正常 2~5 ml)
pH: 7.5 (正常 7.2–7.8)	
精子计数：67×10^6/ml (正常 20~300$\times10^6$/ml)	
精子活力 (在1小时后应有超过50%为活动的精子) 开始时75% 1小时后70%	
精子形态 (应出现少于50%异常形式) 58% 正常形式 42% 异常形式	

41. a. 该结果正常还是异常？
b. 如何指导病人收集标本？
c. 什么是性交后实验？
d. 描述一下阳性和阴性的性交后试验。

a. Is this result normal or abnormal?
b. What instructions would you give for collection?
c. What is a postcoital test?
d. Explain a positive and negative postcoital test.

42. 该患者表现为继发性闭经。
a. 定义继发性闭经。
b. 请将闭经原因按解剖学部位加以分类。
c. 此病人最可能的病因是什么？哪一个部位受影响？
d. 需进行哪些基本检查？

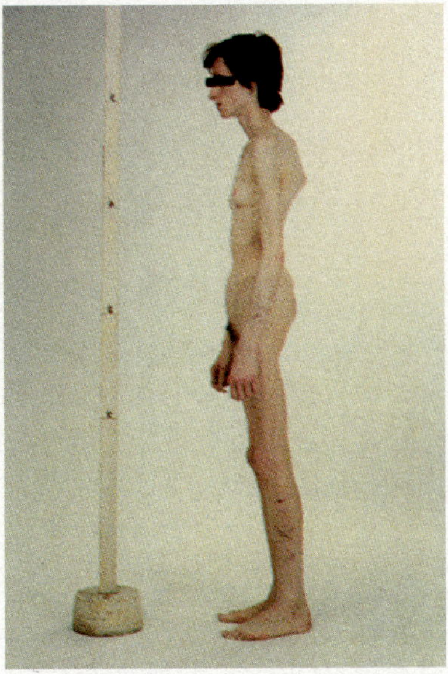

This patient presented with secondary amenorrhoea.
a. Define secondary amenorrhoea.
b. Divide the causes of amenorrhoea into anatomical compartments.
c. What is the likely cause in this patient? What compartment is affected?
d. What baseline investigations would you perform?

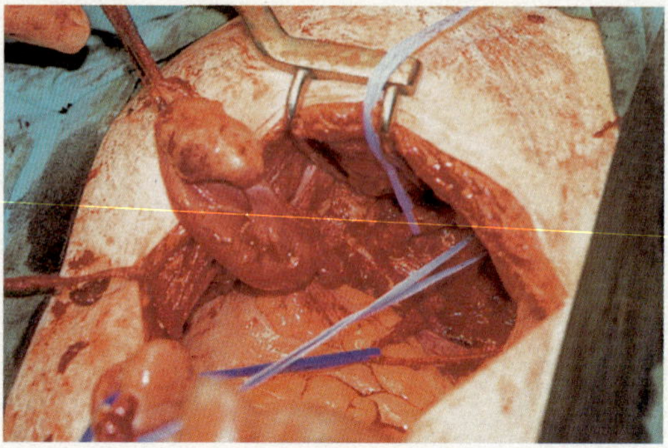

43. 图中所示为 Wertheim 子宫切除术，与 43 题和 44 题有关。
a. 治疗宫颈癌的两种基本方式是什么？
b. 哪些因素可决定治疗方法的选择？
c. 哪些组织被切除？
d. 通过最上方和最下方的带子什么结构被游离出来？

The illustrations in questions 43 and 44 relate to Wertheim's hysterectomy.
a. What two options are available for the first line treatment of cervical carcinoma?
b. What factors determine the choice of treatment?
c. What structures are removed?
d. What structures have been isolated by the uppermost and lowermost tapes?

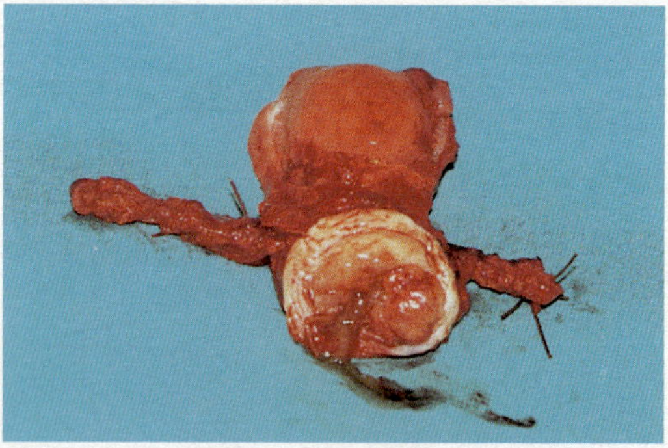

44. a. Wertheim 子宫切除术的适应证是什么？
b. 手术中需对哪些组淋巴结仔细探查？
c. Wertheim 子宫切除术的并发症有哪些？
d. 手术治疗和放疗的相对优点各是什么？

a. What are the indications for a Wertheim's hysterectomy?
b. What lymph node groups are dissected during the procedure?
c. What are the complications of a Wertheim's hysterectomy?
d. What are the relative merits of the surgical approach and radiation therapy?

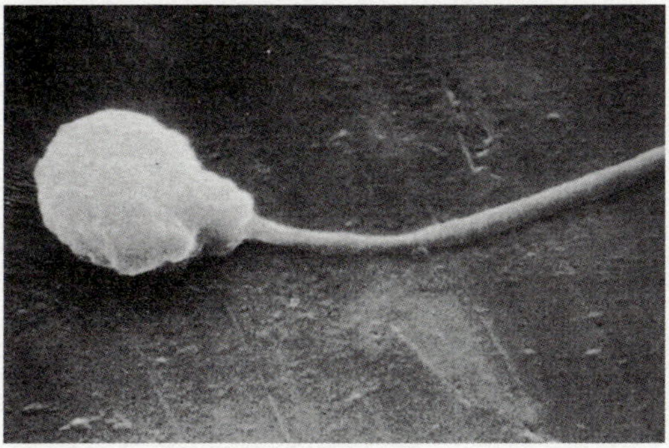

45. a. 电镜下显示的是什么？
b. 其结构由哪些组成？
c. 该结构在哪里产生？
d. 促进其产生的物质是什么？
e. 间质细胞的功能是什么？

a. What does this electron scanning micrograph illustrate?
b. What are the structural components?
c. Where is this structure produced?
d. What is the stimulus for its production?
e. What is the function of the Leydig cells?

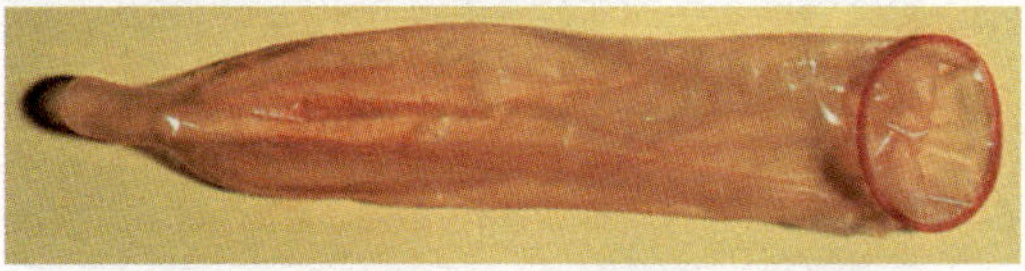

46. a. 使用避孕套避孕的失败率是多少？
b. 描述一下使用和取下避孕套的方法。
c. 该用具的优点是什么？
d. 如果避孕套破了，该如何处理？

a. What is the failure rate of condoms?
b. Describe the method of application and removal.
c. What are the advantages of this device?
d. If this device 'bursts', what is the management?

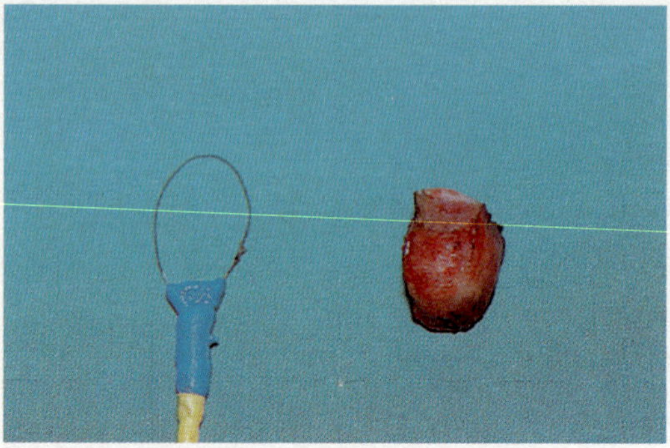

47. a. 该标本和用具的名称是什么?
b. 进行该操作的目的是什么?
c. 进行该操作前应进行何检查?
d. 还可选用其他何种治疗方法?
e. 这一操作的术后并发症是什么? 如何指导病人?

a. What is the name of this specimen and instrument?
b. What is the purpose of this procedure?
c. What investigations should precede this procedure?
d. What alternative procedures are available?
e. What complications can follow this procedure and what advice would you give to the patient?

48. 这是从一个老年妇女腹腔切除的肿物。
a. 该患者可能有何症状?
b. 检查时，何种体征有助于鉴别诊断?
c. 你还要对病人进行何种检查?
d. 如何确诊?
e. 最有可能是什么妇科疾病?

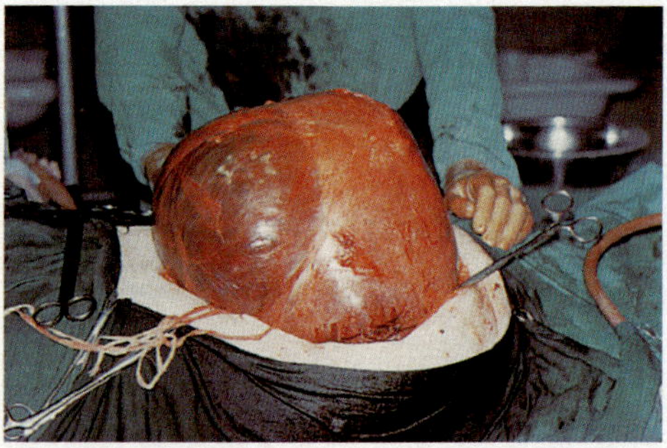

This abdominal mass was removed from an elderly woman.
a. With what symptoms may this woman have presented?
b. On examination, what signs would help with the differential diagnosis?
c. What investigations would you order?
d. How is the definitive diagnosis made?
e. What is the most likely gynaecological diagnosis?

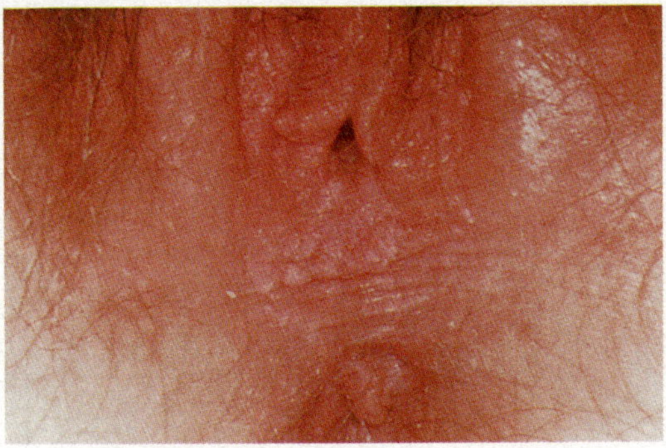

49. a. 该图所示是何疾病?
b. 致病微生物是什么?
c. 此病通常是如何获得的?
d. 治疗模式是什么?
e. 治疗后如何指导患者?

a. What term describes this appearance?
b. What is the aetiological agent?
c. How is this condition usually acquired?
d. What modes of therapy are available?
e. How would you counsel this patient following treatment?

50. 这是手术切除的大网膜。
a. 原发疾病可能是什么?
b. 此原发疾病的主要转移途径是什么?
c. 为何要切除大网膜?
d. 什么因素可影响该病的预后?

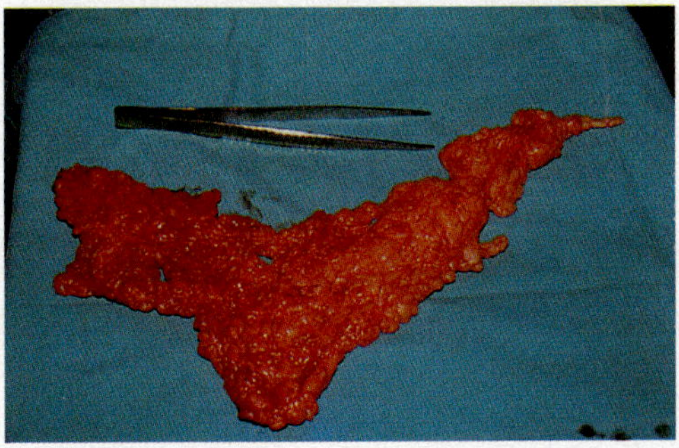

This specimen was removed at omentectomy.
a. What was the likely primary medical condition?
b. What is the typical pattern of spread of the primary condition?
c. Why was the above specimen removed?
d. What factors influence the prognosis of the primary condition?

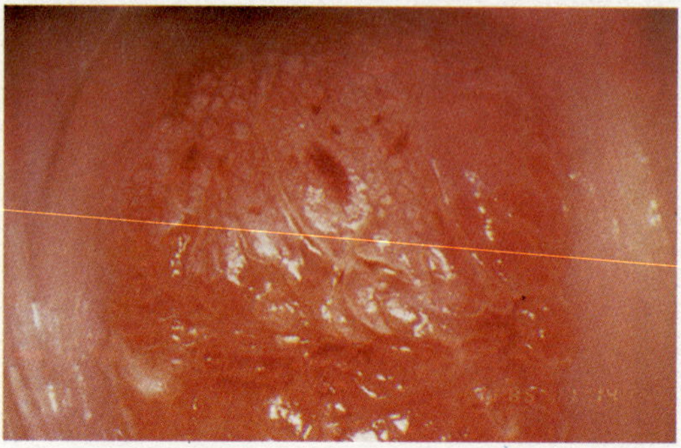

51. 这是经醋酸染色的宫颈。

a. 描述图中所见。

b. 该阴道镜检查提示什么?

c. 如何处理?

d. 该病变能否自发恢复正常?

This cervix has been stained with acetic acid.

a. Describe what you see.

b. What does this colposcopic appearance suggest?

c. What would be your management?

d. Can these changes spontaneously revert to normal?

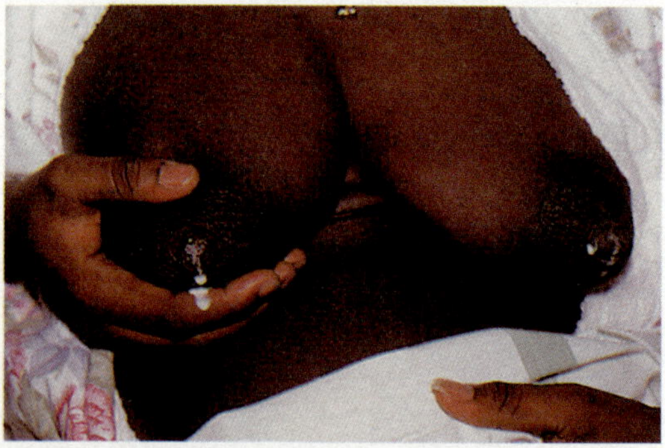

52. a. 描述图中所见。

b. 此为何病?

c. 此病有什么样的妇科表现?

e. 应进行何检查?

a. Describe what you see.

b. What is this condition called?

c. What gynaecological condition may she have presented with?

d. What investigations would you perform?

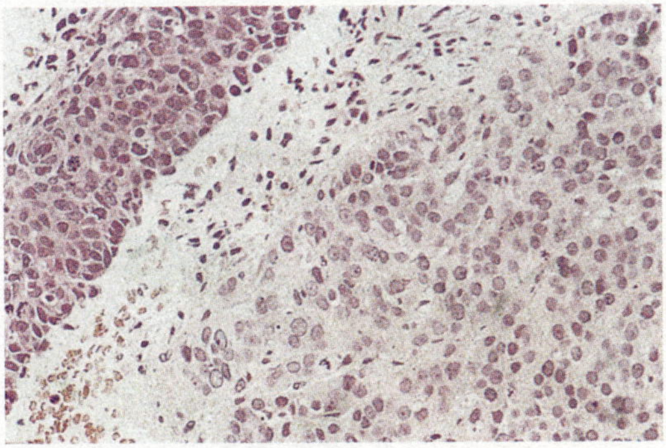

53. 这是一张宫颈切片。

a. 图中可看到什么?

b. 应实施何手术?

c. 该患者绝经后能接受激素替代治疗吗?

This histology slide shows a section of cervix.

a. What can you see?

b. What operation should be performed?

c. Could this woman have HRT when she is postmenopausal?

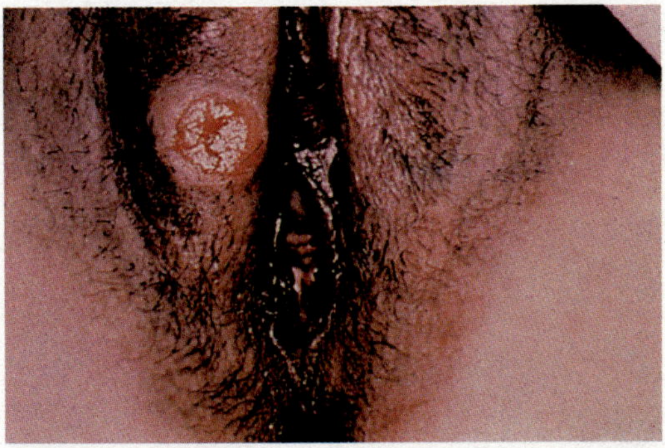

54. a. 诊断为何?

b. 致病微生物是什么?

c. 此病灶在感染后多久可形成?

d. 如何确诊?

e. 此病变如何治疗?

a. What is the diagnosis?

b. Name the causative organism.

c. At what time does the illustrated lesion develop?

d. How is the definitive diagnosis made?

e. How should the illustrated condition be managed?

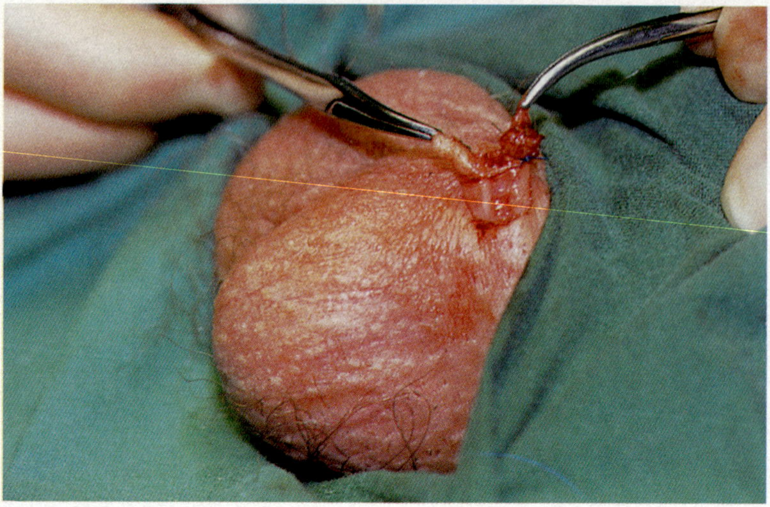

55. a. 游离的是何组织?
b. 手术名称是什么?
c. 术前应向患者交代什么问题?
d. 该手术的并发症是什么?

a. What structure has been isolated?
b. What is the name of this operation?
c. What issues should be discussed in the preoperative counselling?
d. What are the complications of this operation?

56. a. 此操作的性质和目的是什么?
b. 需要何种麻醉方法?
c. 禁忌证是什么?
d. 如何进行操作?
e. 可能出现的不良反应是什么?

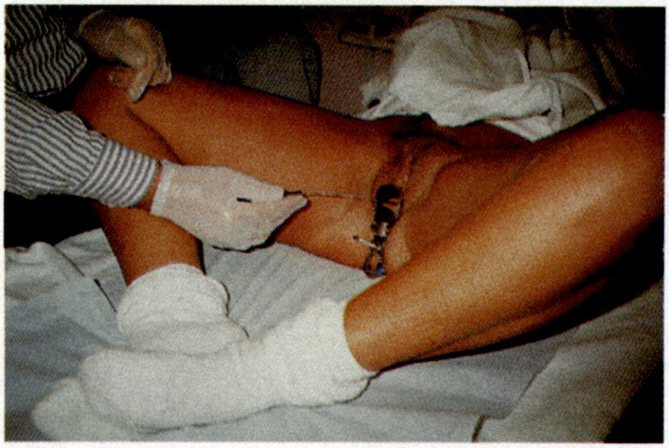

a. What is the nature and purpose of this procedure?
b. What analgesia is required?
c. What are the contraindications?
d. How is this procedure performed?
e. What are the possible adverse reactions?

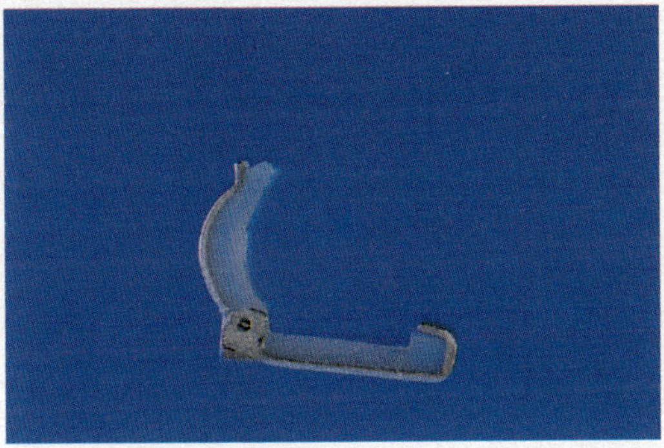

57. a. 这是什么器械?
b. 用途是什么?
c. 进行此操作前应如何向患者交代病情?
d. 失败率是多少?

a. What is this?
b. What is it used for?
c. How would you counsel the patient prior to the procedure?
d. What is the failure rate?

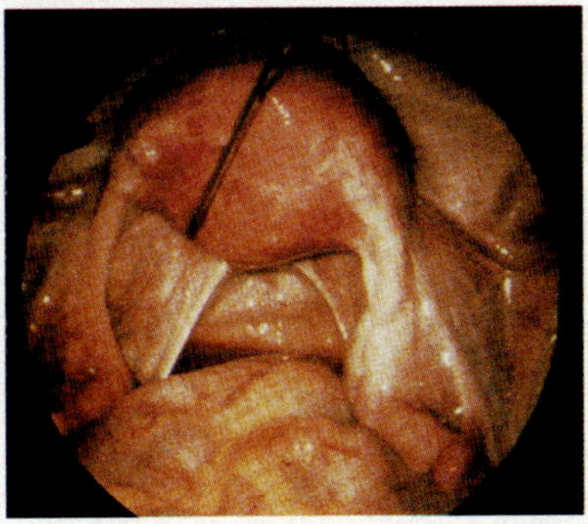

58. a. 此探针支持的是何组织?
b. 在图中心部位像白色带子的结构是什么?
c. 所看到的游离液体一定是病理性的吗?
d. 位于图下 1/3 的结构是什么?

a. What structure is the probe supporting?
b. What are the white band-like structures in the centre portion of the photograph?
c. Is the free fluid that is seen necessarily pathological?
d. What structure occupies the posterior one-third of the illustration?

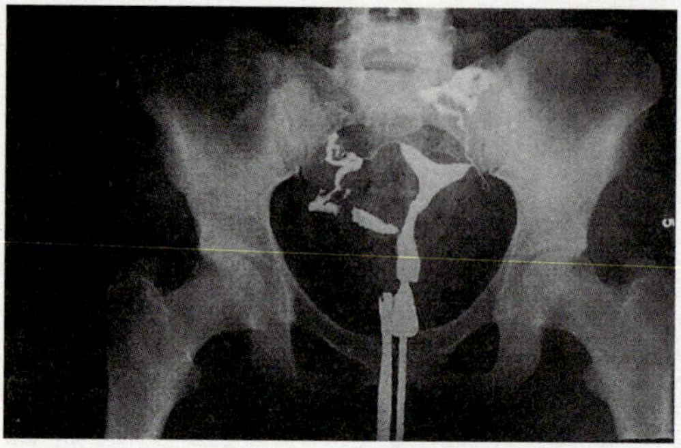

59. a. 此为何种检查?

b. 该检查的适应证是什么?

c. 此操作的风险是什么?

d. 该检查表现为什么?

a. What is the investigation?

b. What are the indications for this investigation?

c. What are the risks of this procedure?

d. What does this investigation show?

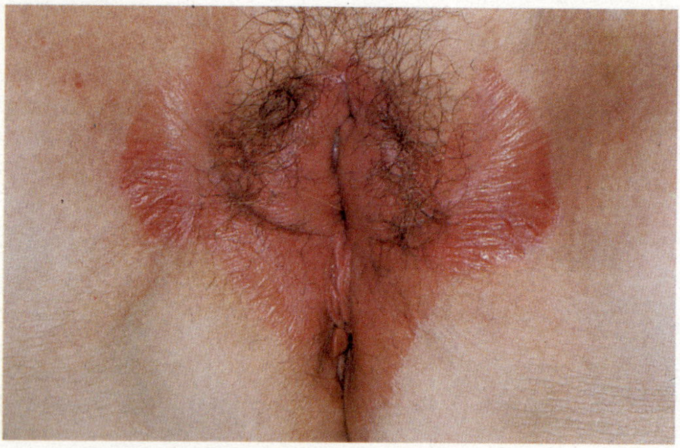

60. 该妇女表现为外阴瘙痒。

a. 可能的病因是什么?

b. 如何诊断?

c. 描述一种该疾病的基本治疗方案。

This woman presented with pruritus vulvae.

a. What are the possible causes?

b. How is the diagnosis made?

c. Describe a typical regime for treatment of the above.

61. a. 正进行何手术?
b. 进行该操作的主要适应证是什么?
c. 与子宫输卵管 X 线造影术相比，该操作的相对优点是什么?
d. 对该患者的输卵管你将发表何意见?

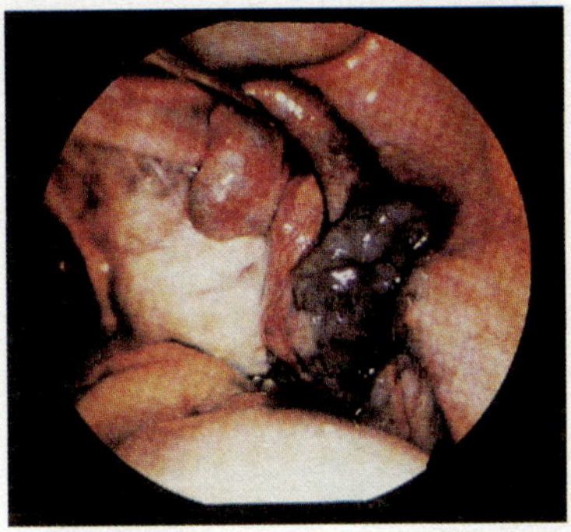

a. What operation has been performed?
b. What are the main indications for this procedure?
c. What are the relative merits for this procedure in comparison to hysterosalpingography?
d. What comment would you make concerning this patient's tubes?

62. 说出a.~e.这5种流产类型。

a.-e. Name the five types of miscarriage.

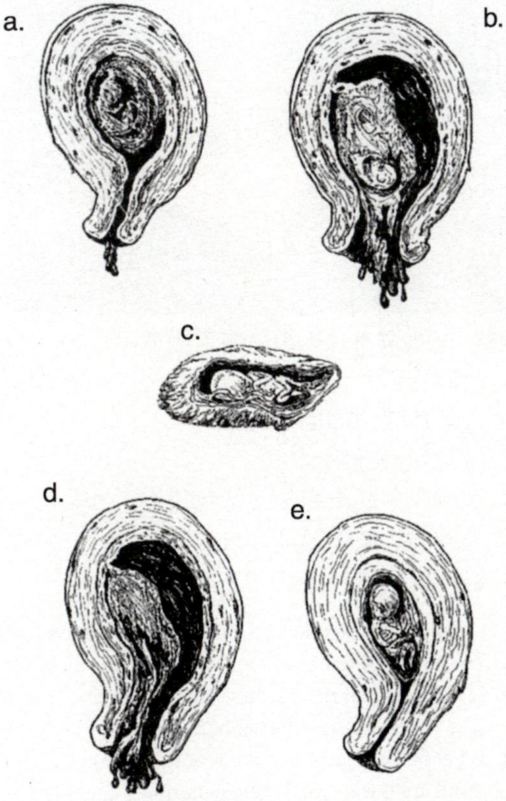

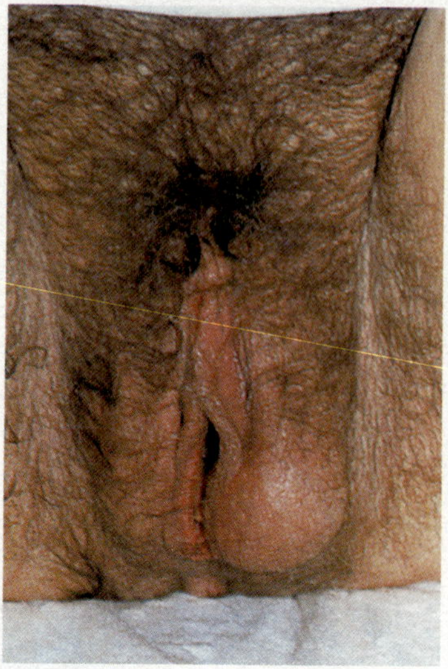

63. a. 描述一下体检所见。
b. 最可能的诊断是什么？
c. 该病灶是如何形成的？
d. 会发生何并发症？
e. 如何处理该患者？

a. Describe the physical findings.
b. What is the most likely diagnosis?
c. How does this lesion form?
d. What complication can occur?
e. How should this patient be managed?

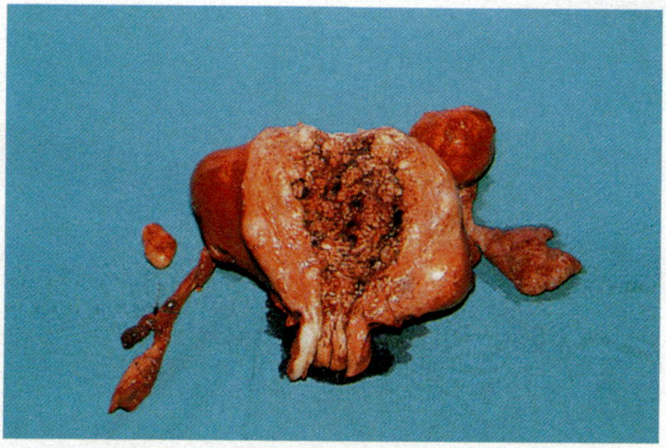

64. 该妇女出现绝经后阴道流血。
a. 诊断为何？
b. 列举出典型的危险因素。
c. 通常如何确诊？
d. 该病典型的组织学类型是什么？
e. 典型的扩散途径是什么？
f. 治疗原则是什么？

This woman presented with postmenopausal bleeding.
a. What is the diagnosis?
b. List the typical risk factors.
c. How is the diagnosis usually confirmed?
d. What is the typical histology of this lesion?
e. What are the characteristic patterns of spread?
f. What are the principles of management?

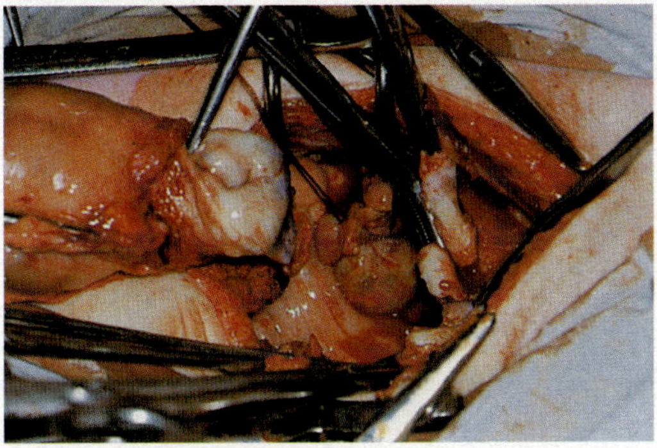

65. a. 正进行何种手术?

b. 该患者卵巢被切除了吗?

c. 哪一结构被染成蓝色?

d. 应用何种线来扎?

a. What operation is being performed?

b. Have the ovaries been removed?

c. What structure is stained blue?

d. What suture has been used to tie the pedicles?

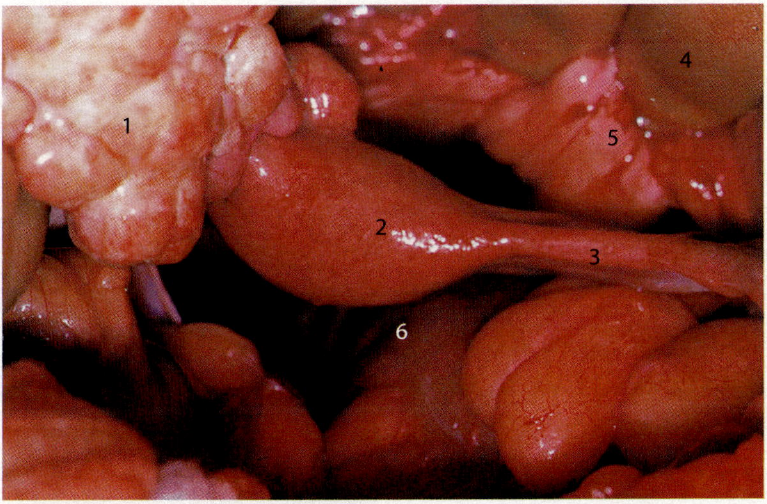

66. 该妇女患左侧卵巢纤维瘤，写出 1 ~ 6 结构的名称。

This woman has a left ovarian fibroma. Name the structures that are numbered 1 to 6.

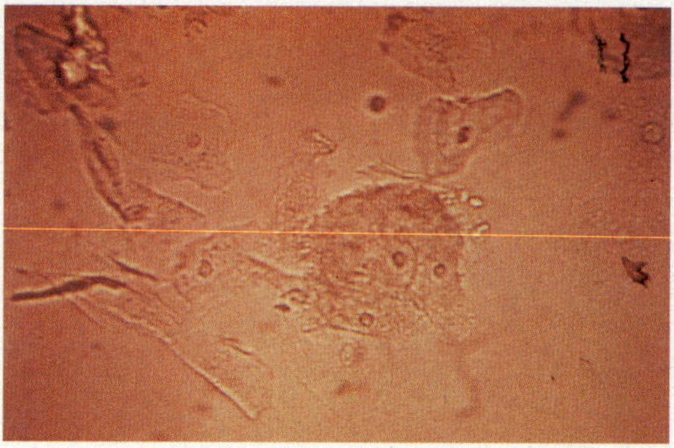

67. a. 引起阴道炎最常见的病因是什么?
b. 革兰染色涂片中的线状物是什么?
c. 该线状物由何组成?
d. 描述特征性的阴道分泌物。
e. 如何治疗?

a. What is the commonest cause of vaginitis?
b. What clue is present in the illustrated Gram stain?
c. What is the composition of the clue?
d. Describe the typical resultant vaginal discharge.
e. How should this vaginitis be treated?

68. 图为肝与前壁腹膜的粘连灶。
a. 这是什么疾病?
b. 病因是什么?
c. 最常见的感染性生物体是什么?
d. 该病有何妇科表现?
e. 如何治疗?

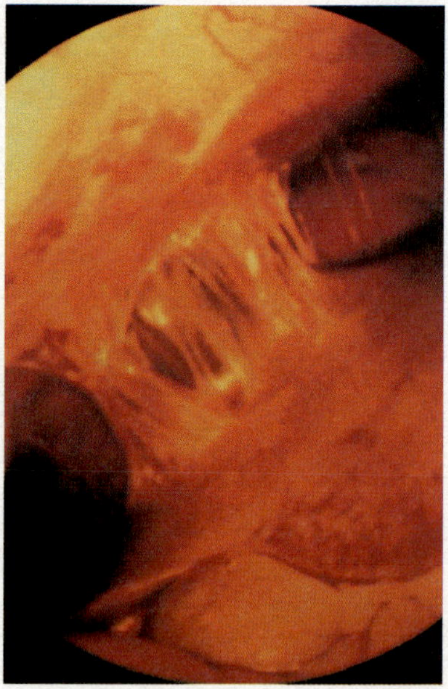

These adhesions were noted between the liver and anterior parietal peritoneum.
a. What is the name of this condition?
b. What is the aetiology?
c. What is the commonest infective organism?
d. How does this condition usually present in gynaecology?
e. What is the treatment?

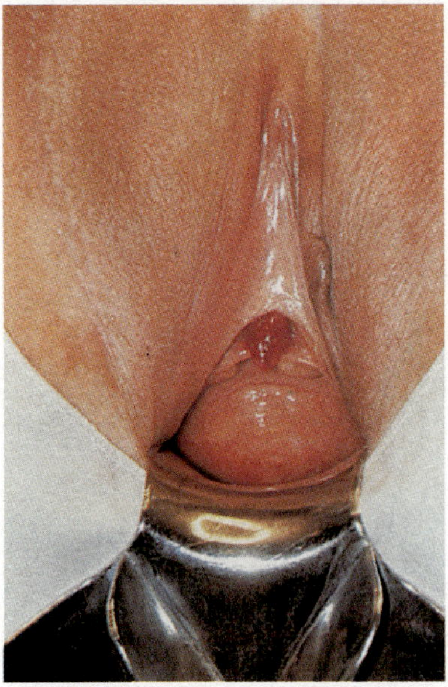

69. a. 膨出的是什么结构?
b. 膨出结构中是何组织?
c. 该患者可能有何症状?
d. 何种手术可纠正这一异常?
e. 尿道有何异常表现?

a. What is the bulging structure?
b. What structure underlies the bulging tissue?
c. With what symptoms may this patient have presented?
d. What operation will correct this abnormality?
e. What urethral abnormality is evident?

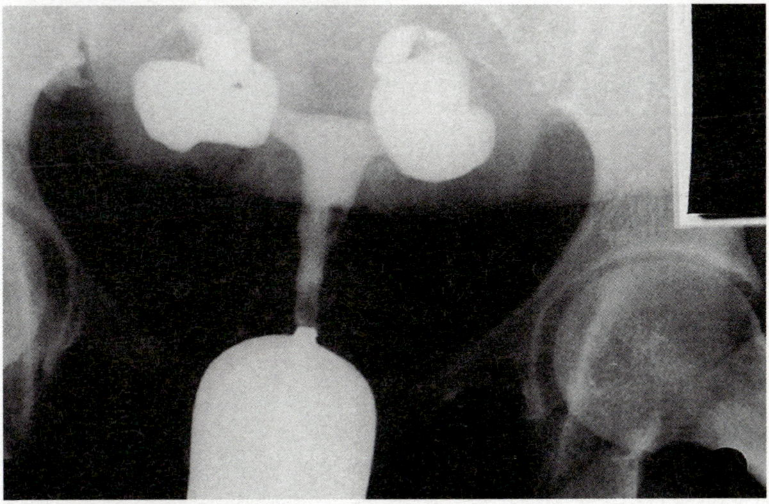

70. a. 该子宫输卵管造影片说明什么?
b. 最可能的病因是什么?
c. 哪一段出现了堵塞?
d. 如该患者主要因不孕就诊，应选择什么治疗?

a. What does this hysterosalpingogram reveal?
b. What is the most likely cause?
c. At what level is the blockage present?
d. If infertility is the patient's main concern, what treatment options are available?

71. a. 正进行何种手术?
b. 支撑子宫的结构是什么?
c. 手术时哪些周围器官和组织易受损?
d. 术后有哪些并发症?

a. What operation is being performed?
b. What are the supporting structures of the uterus?
c. What surrounding structures are at risk of damage during this procedure?
d. What complications can occur postoperatively?

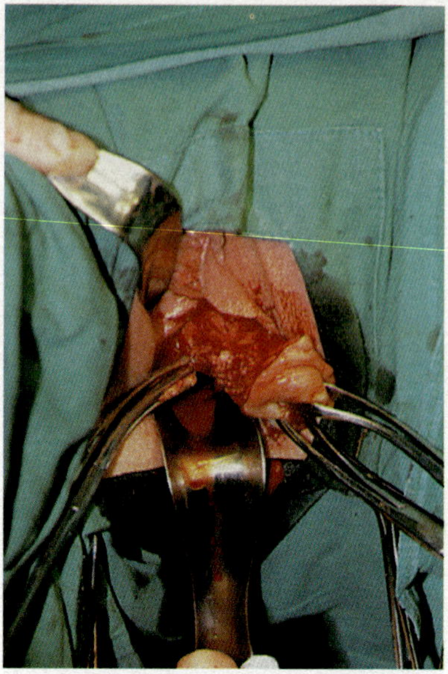

72. 这是绝经后妇女的病灶。
a. 诊断为何?
b. 最可能的症状是什么?
c. 该病灶的主要组织学改变是什么?
d. 如何处理该患者?
e. 如果年轻妇女患此病应如何治疗?

This lesion was present in a postmenopausal woman.
a. What is the diagnosis?
b. What is the most likely presenting symptom?
c. What is the typical histology of this lesion?
d. How would you manage this patient?
e. How would you manage this lesion in a young woman?

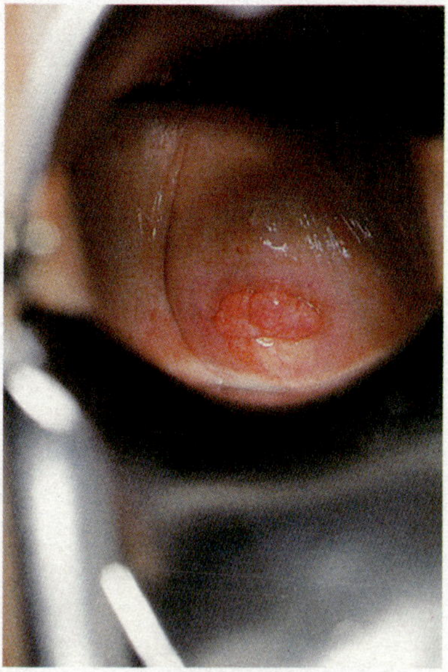

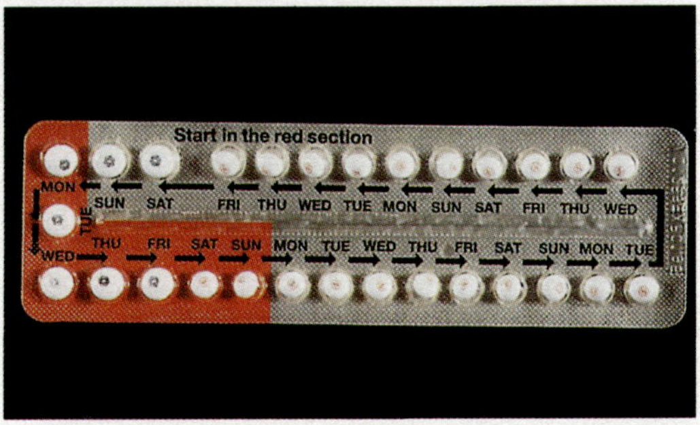

73. a. 这些药片的用途是什么?

b. 除了大一些的药片外，其余的药片成分是什么?

c. 除了显著的优点外，请说出该治疗其他四个优点。

d. 如果病人忘服了最后 2 片红色的药片，可建议她怎么办?

e. 列出此药的两个绝对禁忌证。

a. What are these pills used for?

b. What do these pills (excluding the larger pills) contain?

c. Apart from the obvious benefit of this medication, name four other benefits.

d. If a woman missed the last two pills in the red section, what would you advise her to do?

e. Name two absolute contraindications to this preparation.

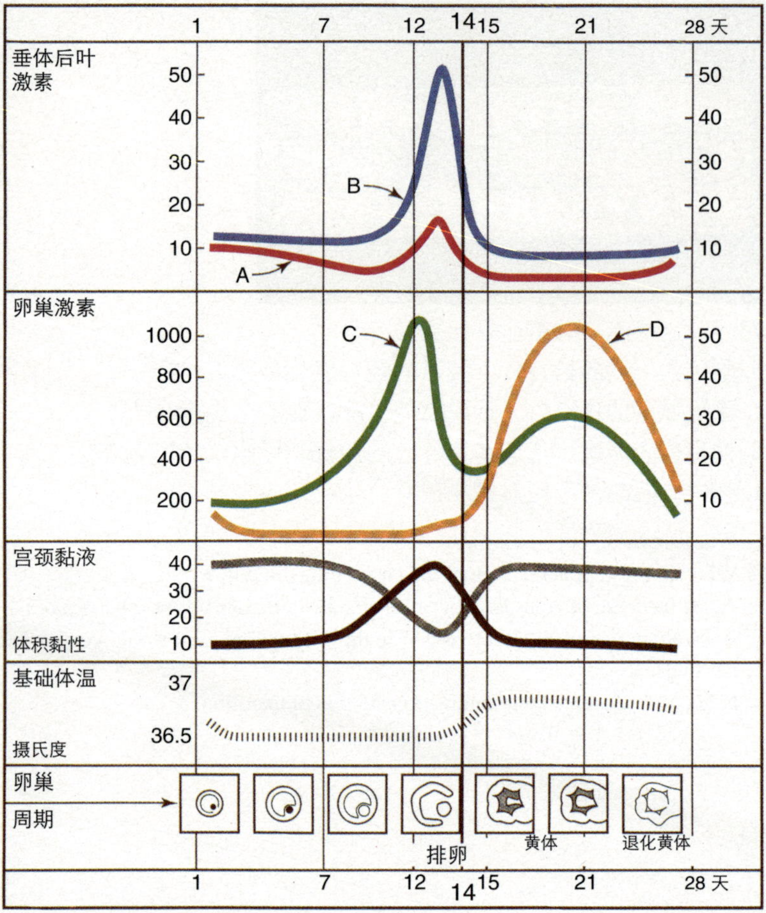

74. a. 请说出这四种激素的名称。

b. 哪两种细胞参与了“C”的合成?

c. 哪些细胞可合成“D”?

d. “D”对宫颈黏液有何影响?

e. 哪种激素引起图中的体温上升?

f. 出生时有多少卵母细胞?

a. Name the four hormones.

b. What two types of cells are involved in the synthesis of C?

c. What cells produce D?

d. What effect does D have on cervical mucus?

e. What hormone causes the temperature rise illustrated?

f. At birth, how many oocytes are present?

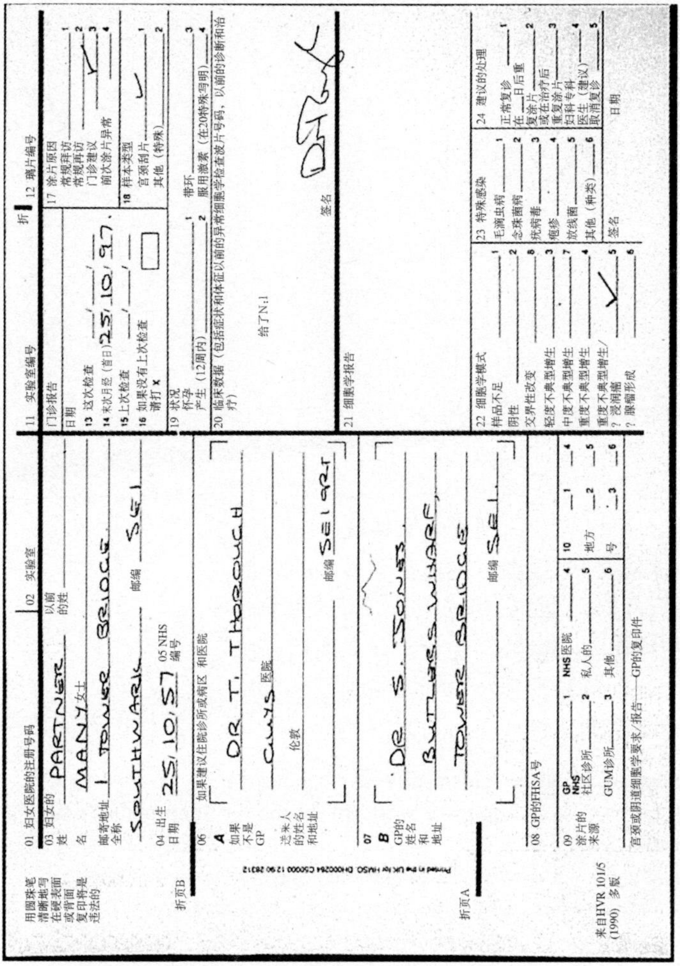

75. a. 此妇女可能有哪些典型症状？说出两个。

b. 看到这个报告你会怎么做？

c. 如果确诊为 Ib，如何治疗？

d. 说出此病的 4 个危险因素。

e. I 期患者的 5 年生存率是多少？

f. 此病的高发年龄组是什么？

a. What classic symptoms may this woman have presented with? Name two.

b. As her GP, what would you do after receiving this report?

c. If the diagnosis is confirmed and is stage 1b, what is the appropriate treatment?

d. Name four risk factors for this disease.

e. What is the 5-year survival for stage 1 disease?

f. What age group has the highest incidence of this disease?

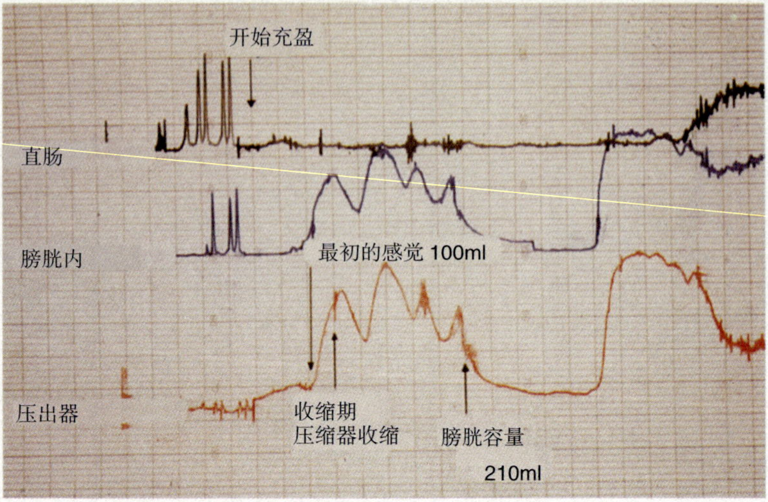

76. a. 什么是尿失禁，列举两个特征。

b. 图为一段膀胱测压图。说出该图显示的异常。

c. 有此检查结果的妇女有何表现？列举两个症状。

d. 有哪些简便方法可减轻症状？列举两种方法。

e. 哪一类药物可能有效？

f. 举例说明此类药物（药名及常用剂量）。

a. Define urinary incontinence. Specify two features.

b. A subtraction cystometric trace is shown. Name the abnormality which is demonstrated.

c. How may a woman with this result present? Specify two symptoms.

d. What simple measures may improve symptoms? Specify two.

e. Which class of drugs may be of benefit?

f. Give an example of this class of drug (generic name with usual dose).

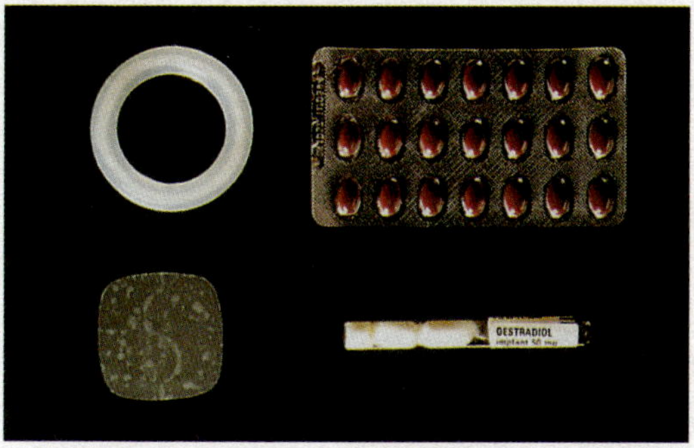

77. 此图为一些常见的药剂。

a. 该组药属于哪类药?

b. 列出这种治疗的绝对禁忌证。

c. 此药物治疗的远期优点是什么? 列举 2 个。

d. 对于有子宫的妇女，除口服孕激素外还可选择哪些给药方式? 列举两种给药方式。

e. 何谓快速耐药性?

f. 采用皮下埋植时，如何减轻快速耐药性?

The photograph shows some commonly used preparations.

a. What is the generic term given to this group of preparations?

b. List two absolute contraindications to this treatment.

c. What are the long-term unseen benefits of such treatment? Name two.

d. In the non-hysterectomised woman, what are the alternatives to oral progestogen? Name two routes of administration.

e. What is meant by tachyphylaxis?

f. When using implants, how might you reduce tachyphylaxis?

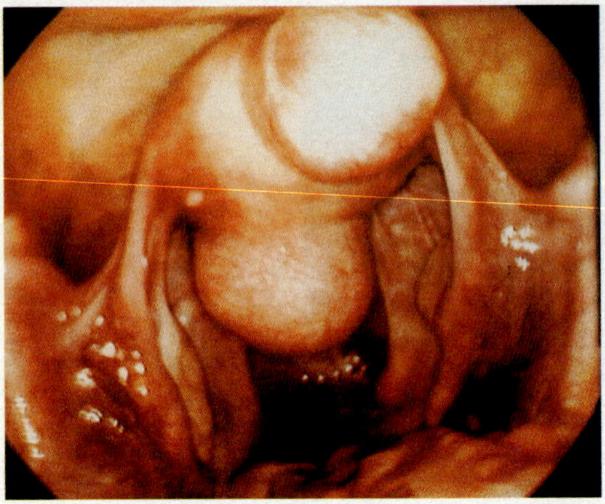

78. 此图是腹腔镜下拍摄的。

a. 显示何种异常?

b. 列出患者可表现的三种症状。

c. 如采用保守手术方法切除病灶，能产生何种术中并发症? 列举两种。

d. 术前应告知患者手术有何危险?

e. 如术前患者已怀孕，请说出她妊娠中的两个并发症。

f. 此病变为恶性的百分比是多少?

This photograph was taken laparoscopically.

a. What abnormality does it show?

b. Name three symptoms this patient may have presented with?

c. If she was to have this abnormality removed by a conservative procedure, what intraoperative complications may arise? Name two.

d. What must a patient be warned about prior to this operation?

e. If this woman had become pregnant prior to her operation, name two complications that she may have had during the pregnancy.

f. In what percentage of cases may this condition be malignant?

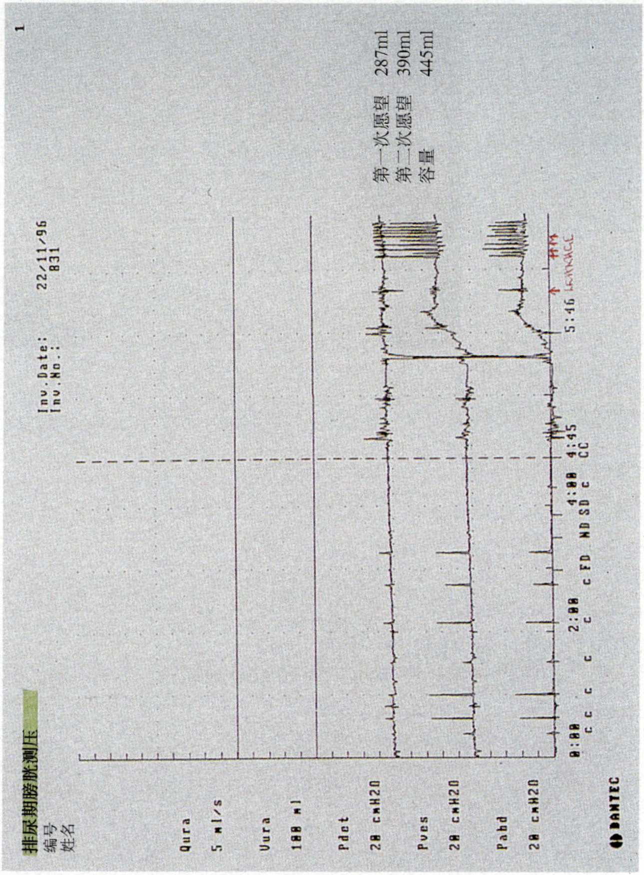

79. a. 根据图示结果，写出检查的名称。

b. 请说出妇女的正常尿流速。

c. 图示有何异常?

d. 哪些简单方法可减轻患者症状? 说出 2 种。

e. 列举出该病的手术治疗方法，并分别举例说明。

f. 已证实的成功率最高的术式是哪种?

g. 对于有经验的医师来说，通常提到的成功率是多少?

a. Look at the result shown. Name the investigation.

b. Define a normal urinary flow rate for a woman.

c. What is the abnormality shown?

d. What simple measures may improve the patient's symptoms? Name two.

e. List three surgical approaches to treat this condition, and provide an example of each.

f. Which operation has the highest documented success rate?

g. What is the usually quoted success rate in experienced hands?

80. 此妇女表现为月经间期出血。

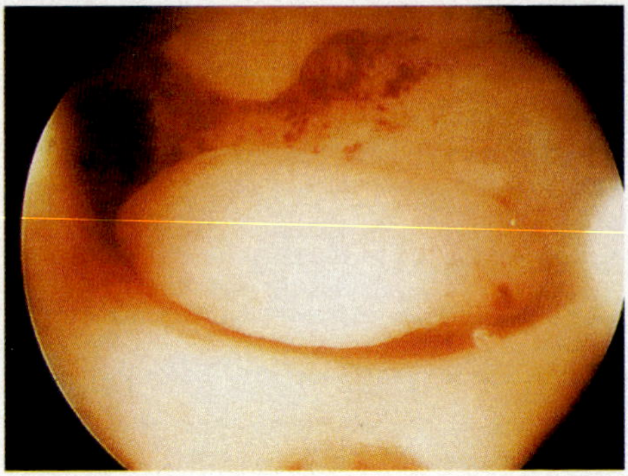

a. 正进行何种手术?
b. 从图中能看到什么?
c. 可进行何种治疗?
d. 月经间期出血的几种其他病因是什么? 说出3种。
e. 可用何种介质来膨胀宫腔? 说出2种。
f. 组织学表现是良性还是恶性?
g. 还可用何种方法来诊断?

This woman presented with IMB.

a. What operation is being performed?
b. What can you see?
c. What management is indicated?
d. What other causes are there for IMB? Name three.
e. What media can be used to distend the cavity? Name two.
f. Is the histology likely to be benign or malignant?
g. How else might this problem have been diagnosed?

81. a. 应用的是何种设备? 可看到什么?

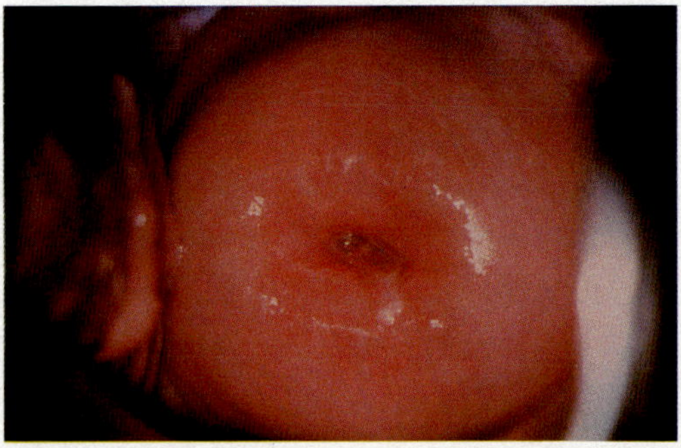

b. 在检查时需用什么溶液?
c. 什么叫核异常?
d. 什么叫发育异常?

a. What instrument is being used here and what does it show?
b. During this investigation what solutions are applied?
c. What is dyskaryosis?
d. What is dysplasia?

1. a. 鳞状上皮细胞。
   b. 细胞核增大、染色质增多及核形不规则。
   c. 建议进行阴道镜检查。

   a. Squamous cells.
   b. Nucleus is enlarged, chromatin is increased and nuclear borders are irregular.
   c. Refer for colposcopy.

2. a. 西姆斯窥器。
   b. 患者取左侧卧位，右腿屈曲，左腿伸直，上方肩膀转向床侧。
   c. 子宫阴道脱垂。用于Cuscoe窥器难以暴露宫颈者。怀疑有瘘管形成。妇科手术。产前阴道流血。
   d. 海绵钳（用于支撑阴道前壁）。

   a. Sims speculum.
   b. The patient is placed in the left lateral position with the right leg bent and the left leg straight. The upper shoulder is rotated towards the bed.
   c. Uterovaginal prolapse. Cases where it is difficult to visualize the cervix with Cuscoe's speculum. Suspected fistulae. In gynaecological operations. Antepartum haemorrhage.
   d. Sponge forceps (to support the anterior vaginal wall).

3. a. 宫内节育器。
   b. 子宫内膜无菌性炎症反应阻碍了孕卵着床，同时改变了精子移动和卵子输送的速率。
   c. 诊断不明的生殖道流血、妊娠、盆腔感染、较大的组织畸形和Wilson病（含铜节育器可引发）。
   d. 无菌术、子宫探子、宫颈钳钳夹宫颈前唇、节育器放置于宫腔内至宫底、剪去尾丝。
   e. 早期并发症：腹痛、迷走神经性休克、子宫穿孔。晚期并发症：感染、流血、节育器脱落和性交痛。
   f. 每5年更换一次。

   a. Intrauterine contraceptive devices.
   b. Endometrial sterile inflammatory reaction that inhibits

implantation. Sperm migration and ovum transport are altered.

c. Undiagnosed genital tract bleeding, pregnancy, pelvic infection, major structural abnormalities and Wilson's disease (copper devices).

d. Aseptic technique, uterus sounded, anterior lip of the cervix is grasped with a volsellum forceps and the device is inserted in the uterine cavity to the predetermined length and the strings are cut.

e. Immediate complications: pain, vasovagal shock, uterine perforation. Late complications: infection, menorrhagia, expulsion and male dyspareunia.

f. Every 5 years.

4. a. 念珠菌感染（鹅口疮）。

b. 瘙痒和阴道分泌物。

c. 微生物拭子。

d. 抗真菌药物如克霉唑或益康唑。

e. 确诊后，夫妻双方应同时治疗。女性患者应用强效的口服药，如氟康唑。

a. Candidal infection (thrush).

b. Itching and vaginal discharge.

c. Microbiological swab.

d. Antifungal agents such as clotrimazole or econazole.

e. After positively confirming the diagnosis, both partners should be treated concomitantly. The female partner should be treated with a powerful oral agent such as fluconazole.

5. a. 细胞内革兰染色阴性的双球菌。

b. 淋病。

c. 尿道炎、易逆行感染至上生殖道的宫颈炎，也可发生肛门直肠和咽部的感染。淋菌败血症性关节炎通常累及膝部。

d. 细菌培养中证实有病原体。

e. 除外并发感染，适当的抗生素治疗，治疗期间应禁止性生活，追踪性生活史，并对其治疗进行随访。

a. Gram-negative intracellular diplococci.

b. Gonorrhoea.

c. Urethritis, cervicitis which may ascend into the upper genital tract, anorectal and pharyngeal infection. Septic gonococcal arthritis usually involves the knee.

d. Demonstration of the organism in culture.

e. Exclude concomitant infection, appropriate antibiotic therapy, cessation of sex during treatment, tracing of sexual contacts, follow-up for test-of-cure.

6. a. 女性生殖器官阉割。
   b. 排尿困难、痛经和性交困难。
   c. 宫颈扩张困难和分娩时出口梗阻。
   d. 阴唇成形术。
   e. 会阴前端切开术。

   a. Female genital mutilation (FGM).
   b. Difficulty with micturition, painful menstruation and dyspareunia.
   c. Difficulty with cervical assessment and obstructed labour at the outlet.
   d. Labioplasty - reversal of the FGM.
   e. Anterior episiotomy.

7. a. 可见垂体窝扩大和双底边。
   b. CT、MRI。
   c. 垂体微腺瘤。继发闭经、不孕和溢乳。
   d. 血清泌乳素、视野和甲状腺功能测定以及垂体窝 CT 检查。
   e. 药物（如吩噻嗪、灭吐灵、甲基多巴），其他的垂体和下丘脑肿瘤，原发的甲状腺功能减退和妊娠。
   f. 卡麦角林、垂体切除术和放疗。

   a. Enlargement of the pituitary fossa and double flooring of the fossa.
   b. CT, MRI.
   c. Pituitary adenoma. Secondary amenorrhoea, infertility and galactorrhoea.
   d. Serum prolactin, visual fields and thyroid function tests, CT of the fossa.
   e. Drugs (e.g. phenothiazines, metoclopramide, methyldopa), other pituitary and hypothalamic tumours, primary hypothyroidism, pregnancy.
   f. Carbergoline, hypophysectomy, and radiation therapy.

8. a. 宫颈涂片检查。可用来筛查异常宫颈上皮细胞。
   b. Aylesbury 铲型刮勺。
   c. 正常每隔 3 年查一次。
   d. 移行带。

e. 应快速制作涂片，且无血迹，在载玻片上涂片（应薄而均匀）并且需立即固定。

a. Cervical smear test. This is a screening test to detect abnormal cervical cells.
b. Aylesbury spatula.
c. Normal recall is 3-yearly.
d. Transformation zone.
e. The smear must be taken quickly, in the absence of blood, smeared (thinly and evenly) across a glass slide and fixed immediately.

9. a. 外阴癌。
b. 绝经后妇女。
c. 鳞状细胞癌。
d. 经淋巴转移到腹股沟深、浅淋巴结和股深淋巴结，然后达髂外淋巴结，可直接浸润到阴道、尿道和肛门。
e. 根治性切除术，包括整块切除两侧回流的淋巴结。

a. Vulval carcinoma.
b. Postmenopausal women.
c. Squamous cell carcinoma.
d. Lymphatic spread to the superficial and deep inguinal and femoral nodes and then to the external iliac nodes. Direct spread occurs to vagina, urethra and anus.
e. Radical excision with en bloc dissection of the draining nodes on both sides.

10. a. 基础体温表。
b. 在第 14 天体温略有下降，随后体温上升了 0.6℃并持续了 12 天，性交的时间看来较适宜。
c. 有排卵。
d. 第 21 天的孕酮值（周期为 28 天）。

a. Basal body temperature chart.
b. There is a small drop in the temperature on day 14, followed by a rise in the temperature of approximately 0.6℃ that persists for 12 days. Timing of intercourse appears to have been appropriate.
c. Ovulation.
d. Day 21 progesterone (in a 28-day cycle).

11. a. 宫内假孕囊，右附件区可见孕囊。
b. 闭经后出现下腹痛及阴道流血（典型者约 6 周左右）伴肩部

疼痛。

c. 一侧腹部触痛，子宫小于停经日数，宫口关闭，一侧附件区触痛和宫颈刺激症，且可扪及较柔软的附件包块。

d. 血 β -HCG 监测和腹腔镜。

a. Uterine pseudogestational sac, true gestational sac containing a fetus in the right adnexum.

b. Low abdominal pain with vaginal bleeding after amenorrhoea (classically about 6 weeks), shoulder-tip pain.

c. Unilateral abdominal tenderness, uterine size less than dates, cervical os closed, unilateral adnexal tenderness and cervical excitation, a tender adnexal mass.

d. Serial quantitative beta-HCG levels and laparoscopy.

12. a. 先天输卵管发育异常、盆腔炎、输卵管手术史、宫内节育器、既往宫外孕史和辅助生殖技术史。

b. 输卵管壶腹部、输卵管其他部位、卵巢、阔韧带、宫颈和腹腔。

c. 输卵管流产、腹腔内出血，可能出现输卵管破裂和极少见的腹腔妊娠甚至达妊足月。

d. 其他的早孕并发症、盆腔炎、卵泡破裂、黄体出血和阑尾炎。

a. Congenital tubal abnormalities, pelvic inflammatory disease, tubal surgery, intrauterine contraceptive devices, previous ectopic pregnancy and assisted conception techniques.

b. Ampulla, other portions of the tube, ovary, broad ligament, cervix and abdominal cavity.

c. Tubal abortion, pelvic haematocele, possible tubal rupture and rarely an abdominal pregnancy that progresses to term.

d. Other complications of early pregnancy, pelvic inflammatory disease, ovarian cyst accidents, bleeding from the corpus luteum and appendicitis.

13. a. 全身化疗、腹腔镜手术（输卵管切开术、输卵管切除术或注射胚胎毒性物质）、开腹手术（线性输卵管切开术、部分切除术和输卵管切除术）、保守治疗（监测HCG水平和临床体征）。

b. 初始病变很可能是双侧的，悲伤/哀丧咨询可能是需要的，再次妊娠需早期行超声检查。

c. 再发风险由对侧输卵管的情况而定。大约在10% ~ 15%之间。

a. Systemic chemotherapy, laparoscopic techniques (salpingostomy salpingectomy or injection of embryotoxic substances), open laparotomy (linear salpingostomy, segmental resection, salpingectomy).

Conservative management - monitoring BHCG levels and clinical signs.

b. The original pathology is probably bilateral. Grief/bereavement counselling may be required. An early ultrasound scan is required in future pregnancies.

c. Risk is determined by the condition of the contralateral tube. Varies between 10% and 15%.

14. 宫颈癌和子宫内膜癌。

a. 外放射治疗、近距治疗（放射源贴近目标）和腔内治疗。

b. 皮肤红斑、脱发、尿急、尿频、恶心、呕吐、腹痛、里急后重、腹泻和骨髓抑制。

c. 直肠炎、直肠阴道瘘、肠管轻微受损可引起吸收不良和狭窄形成、出血性膀胱炎、不孕和阴道狭窄。继发的恶性疾病偶可发生。

a. Carcinoma of the cervix and endometrium.

b. External beam radiation therapy, brachytherapy (source close to target), intracavitary.

c. Skin erythema and hair loss, urinary urgency and frequency, nausea and vomiting, abdominal pain, tenesmus, diarrhoea and bone marrow suppression.

d. Proctitis, rectovaginal fistula, small bowel injury with malabsorption and stricture formation, haemorrhagic cystitis, sterility and vaginal stenosis. Secondary malignancies may occasionally be seen.

15. a. 子宫内膜异位症，指子宫内膜组织异位到宫腔以外的部位。

b. 体腔上皮化生，经血逆流，继发种植，经静脉或淋巴播散。

c. 症状是继发性痛经、性交痛、慢性盆腔痛和不孕。体征包括盆腔触痛、有或无盆腔包块或结节和子宫后倾固定。

d. 病灶活检。

a. Endometriosis. This is defined as endometrial tissue in sites other than the uterine cavity.

b. Coelomic metaplasia, retrograde menstruation and subsequent implantation, venous or lymphatic spread.

c. Symptoms are secondary dysmenorrhoea, dyspareunia, chronic pelvic pain and infertility. Signs include pelvic tenderness, ± pelvic masses or nodules, and fixed retroversion of the uterus.

d. Biopsy of the lesion.

16. a. 此妇女表现为乳房发育良好，但无阴道。

b. 睾丸女性化。

c. 该女性染色体核型是46, YX且对雄激素不敏感。

d. 通常在青春期后有乳房发育和原发性闭经。

e. 无腋毛或腋毛稀少，外阴发育正常，缺乏宫颈的短盲管状阴道。无子宫。可在腹腔内、腹股沟内或偶尔在阴唇内发现睾丸。

a. The person illustrated has good breast development but no pubic hair.

b. Testicular feminization.

c. The person is a 46,XY individual with androgen insensitivity.

d. Usually after puberty with normal breast development and primary amenorrhoea.

e. Absent or scanty axillary hair, normal vulva, short blind vagina with no cervix. Absent uterus. Testes are found in either the abdomen, the groins or occasionally the labia.

17. a. 该手术标本显示了子宫、双侧输卵管卵巢和一个子宫内膜息肉。

b. 通常无症状，也可出现不正常的阴道流血和绝经后流血。如息肉脱出宫颈外，会导致痛经或性交后出血。

c. 可直接检查发现。在宫腔镜检查时可直接看到。诊刮时可通过器械感觉到，超声检查也可检测到。

d. 可用息肉钳钳夹出，但理想的方法是通过宫腔镜手术切除，也可采用子宫切除术。

a. Surgical specimen showing uterus, tubes and ovaries and an endometrial polyp.

b. No symptoms, abnormal vaginal bleeding, postmenopausal bleeding. If they protrude through the cervix they may cause dysmenorrhoea or postcoital bleeding.

c. May be detected on visual examination. At hysteroscopy they will be seen directly, and at D&C they may be felt with an instrument. An ultrasound scan may also detect them.

d. They may be removed using polyp forceps but ideally they should be resected with an operating hysteroscope. Hysterectomy is an option.

18. a. 主要作用机制是抑制排卵，还作用于子宫内膜和宫颈黏液水平以及输卵管，对避孕起补充作用。
    b. 不。起初予以高剂量，随后减少剂量。
    c. 很少失败。
    d. 效果好而且方便，减少了大出血、贫血、痛经、经前紧张状态和内异症的发病率。
    e. 易发生突破性出血、恢复受孕延迟、体重增加、溢乳和轻微的雄激素影响。

    a. The primary action is to prevent ovulation, and this is supplemented by contraceptive actions at the endometrial and mucus levels and also in the fallopian tube.
    b. No. There is a high level initially, which declines thereafter.
    c. Failure rarely occurs.
    d. Highly effective and convenient; diminished incidence of heavy bleeding, anaemia, dysmenorrhoea, premenstrual tension symptoms, endometriosis.
    e. Breakthrough bleeding, delay in the return of fertility, weight gain, galactorrhoea and mild androgenic effects.

19. a. 阴道镜检查。
    b. 宫颈涂片异常，孕妇在妊娠期间摄入己烯雌酚后所分娩的女孩，怀疑有阴道或外阴的上皮内瘤样病变。
    c. 可通过双瓣的窥器暴露宫颈。把醋酸涂于宫颈表面，然后进行观察。阴道镜直视下可取材进行活检。
    d. 应向患者详细说明检查的必要性，如果不考虑为浸润性癌，也应说清楚。解释操作过程时不应使用医学术语。如果涂片结果提示有疣病毒的存在，需对此病原体的性传播特性予以说明。目前的性伴侣也需进行检查。而与以后的性伴侣性交需带避孕套。

    a. Colposcopy.
    b. Abnormal smear, female offspring of women who ingested stilboestrol antenatally, suspicion of vaginal/vulval intraepithelial neoplasia.
    c. The cervix is viewed with a bivalve speculum. Acetic acid is

applied to the cervix, which is then inspected. A colposcopically directed biopsy is usually taken.

d. The need for the examination should be explained and, if there is no suspicion of invasive cancer, this should be clearly stated. An explanation of the procedure should be given in nonmedical terms. If the smear result has revealed the presence of wart virus, the sexually transmissible nature of this organism needs to be discussed. The current partner may also need to be checked, and condoms should be worn with any future new partners.

20. a. 平滑肌瘤。

b. 月经过多、痛经、腹部胀满、尿频。

c. 促性腺激素释放激素激动剂。

a. Fibroids.

b. Menorrhagia, dysmenorrhoea, distended abdomen, urinary frequency.

c. Gonadotrophin-releasing hormone analogues.

21. a. 病史：症状发作与持续时间，青春期发育情况和月经史，家族史和用药史。

体检：体重，血压，男性化的体征，多毛或常见的内分泌病，阴道检查。

辅助检查：血清游离睾酮检测，由病史和体检所示应进行的其他性激素检查，盆腔超声检查，如临床需要可行肾上腺CT以及腹腔镜检查。

b. 右侧卵巢有一可产生雄激素的肿瘤。

c. 男性细胞瘤（支持细胞和/或间质细胞瘤）、脂质细胞瘤、门细胞瘤以及偶发的卵巢转移性肿瘤。

d. 除了声音粗哑以外，其他的症状都可消退。

a. History: onset and duration of symptoms, pubertal and menstrual history, family history and medication intake.

Examination: weight, blood pressure, signs of virilism, hirsutism or general endocrinopathy, vaginal examination.

Investigations: serum free testosterone, other appropriate hormone assays as suggested by the history and examination, pelvic (ovarian) ultrasound and, if clinically indicated, CT scan of adrenal glands, laparoscopy.

b. An androgen-producing tumour of the right ovary.

c. Androblastomas (Sertoli cell and/or Leydig cell tumours), lipoid cell tumours, hilar cell tumours and occasionally metastatic tumours of the ovaries.

d. All signs regress apart from deepening of the voice.

22. a. 生殖器疱疹。

b. 疼痛、性交痛、排尿困难、红斑、水肿、小囊泡、疼痛性溃疡和腹股沟淋巴结病。

c. 确诊，后入院，止痛，如有需要可行导管插入麻醉，主要行局麻，治疗继发感染。尽早应用阿昔洛韦。对患者解释诊断和病史。

d. 如分娩时疱疹处于活动期，而且胎膜未破或胎膜已破未超过 4 小时，可行剖宫产结束分娩。

a. Herpes genitalis.

b. Pain, dyspareunia, dysuria, erythema, oedema, vesicles, painful ulcers, inguinal lymphadenopathy.

c. Confirm diagnosis, admit to hospital, analgesia, catheterization if required, topical local anaesthetic, treatment of secondary infection. Aciclovir can help if commenced early. Explanation of the diagnosis and the natural history.

d. If a woman with active herpes presents in labour, delivery by caesarean section is indicated if the membranes are intact or have been ruptured for less than 4 hours.

23. a. 宫颈癌。

b. 平均年龄是 52 岁，两个高发年龄段分别为 35 ~ 39 岁和 60 ~ 64 岁。

c. 月经间期出血或性交后及绝经后出血和异常阴道分泌物。

d. 直接蔓延到邻近组织（如阴道、宫体和子宫旁组织），还有淋巴和血行转移。

e. 需检查颈部和腹股沟淋巴结，胸部X片和静脉注射肾盂照影。麻醉下检查（腹腔镜检查、直肠阴道双合诊检查、宫颈活检和诊刮等）。其他检查如全身骨骼 X 片和直肠镜检查。

f. 分期：Ⅰ期：癌症局限于宫颈。

Ⅱ期：累及阴道的上 2/3 或播散至宫旁但未达盆壁。

Ⅲ期：累及阴道下 1/3 或达盆壁以及所有病例均有肾积水或无功能肾。

Ⅳ期：播散到邻近器官如膀胱或直肠或有远处器官转移。

a. Carcinoma of the cervix.
b. The mean age is 52 years. Bimodal distribution with peaks at 35-39 years and 60-64 years.
c. Intermenstrual, postcoital or postmenopausal bleeding and abnormal vaginal discharge.
d. Direct invasion into surrounding structures (vagina, uterine body, parametrium). Lymphatic and haematogenous metastasis.
e. The neck and groin nodes should be checked. Chest X-ray, intravenous pyelogram, examination under anaesthetic (cystoscopy, bimanual rectovaginal examination, cervical biopsy, D&C). Additional procedures may include a skeletal X-ray and proctoscopy.
f. *Stage 1*: carcinoma confined to the cervix.
Stage 2: spread to either the upper two-thirds of the vagina or the parametrium but without extension to the pelvic side wall.
Stage 3: involvement of the lower third of the vagina, extension to the pelvic side wall and all cases with hydronephrosis or a nonfunctioning kidney.
Stage 4: spread to adjacent structures such as bladder or rectum or spread to distant organs.

24. a. Cuscoe 窥器。
b. 仰卧位。
c. 用左手分开阴唇以便能看到入口，窥器的两叶应合拢并沿顺时针方向插入阴道的后下方，窥器置入后两叶张开宫颈就可暴露出来。
d. 双合诊检查盆腔器官。

a. Cuscoe's.
b. Dorsal position.
c. The labia are parted with the left hand in order to visualize the introitus. The speculum is inserted and rotated clockwise with the blades together in a posteroinferior direction. Once the speculum is in place the blades are separated and the cervix is visualized between the blades.
d. Bimanual examination to assess the pelvic organs.

25. a. 良性囊性畸胎瘤（皮样囊肿）。
b. 年轻妇女尤其是年龄在 20~30 岁的妇女。
c. 病灶起源于原始生殖细胞，可包括头发、上皮、软骨和骨骼和牙齿，还可见其他组织结构。

d. 为 10%。对侧的卵巢也应检查。
e. 恶性生殖细胞肿瘤很少见，在年轻妇女尤其罕见。

a. Benign cystic teratoma (dermoid).
b. In young females particularly between the ages of 20 and 30 years.
c. This lesion derives from the primary germ cell layers and can contain structures such as hair, epidermis, cartilage, bone and, of course, teeth. Many other structures can also be found.
d. 10%. The contralateral ovary must always be inspected.
e. Malignant germ cell tumours are rare, especially in young females.

26. a. 正常的宫颈柱状上皮。
b. 纳氏囊肿。
c. 不成熟的化生。
d. 原始鳞柱交界部。

a. Normal columnar epithelium.
b. Nabothian follicle.
c. Immature metaplasia.
d. Original squamocolumnar junction.

27. a. 多毛症。
b. Ferriman 和 Gallway 体系，在这一体系中，对全身各部的毛发生长都给予评分。
c. 特发性的、卵巢的（如多囊卵巢综合征、分泌雄激素的肿瘤）、肾上腺的（如库欣综合征、先天性肾上腺增生和分泌雄激素的肿瘤）以及药物等。
d. 测定血清睾酮、黄体生成素、卵泡刺激素和性激素结合球蛋白水平。
e. 让患者放心、局部治疗、漂白剂、拔除汗毛、剔除汗毛、上蜡、电针除毛、药物（口服避孕药、醋酸环丙氯地孕酮、螺内脂）。药物治疗必需至少要达到 18 个月。

a. Hirsutism.
b. The Ferriman and Gallway system, in which various parts of the body are graded for the degree of hair growth.
c. Idiopathic, ovarian (polycystic ovarian syndrome, androgen-producing tumours), adrenal (Cushing's syndrome, congenital adrenal hyperplasia, androgen-secreting tumours), drugs.
d. Serum testosterone, LH, FSH, SHBG.
e. Reassurance, local treatment, bleaching agents, plucking, shaving,

waxing, electrolysis, drugs (oral contraceptive pill, cyproterone acetate, spironolactone). Drug therapy must be for a minimum period of 18 months.

28. a. 子宫托。
    b. 架型、蘑菇型和环型。
    c. 架型和环型的子宫托可用于：子宫脱垂和阴道膨出（患者拒绝或不适合行手术）者；当等待手术或者为了帮助褥疮溃疡恢复；妊娠者。蘑菇型宫托：可用于使后倾的子宫前倾前屈。
    d. 阴道分泌物，溃疡形成，阴道流血，不舒适感，久置不取可引起嵌顿。
    e. 应4～6个月更换一次。

    a. Pessaries.
    b. Shelf, Hodge, ring pessary.
    c. Shelf, ring pessary: uterovaginal prolapse (patient declines or is unsuitable for surgery); while awaiting surgery or in order to aid healing of decubitus ulceration; in pregnancy. Hodge pessary: this is used in order to antevert a retroverted uterus.
    d. Vaginal discharge, ulceration, vaginal bleeding, discomfort, impaction if neglected.
    e. 4~6-monthly.

29. a. 腹腔镜检查。
    b. 二氧化碳。
    c. 在腹腔内的任何器官。
    d. 需排空膀胱而且必需在麻醉下进行EUA。

    a. Laparoscopy.
    b. Carbon dioxide.
    c. Any organs that are within the peritoneal cavity.
    d. The bladder must be emptied and an EUA must be performed.

30. a. CIN Ⅲ和正常的鳞状上皮。
    b. 没有。
    c. 每年进行一次涂片检查。
    d. 严重的核异型。

    a. CIN III and normal squamous epithelium.
    b. No.
    c. Yearly smears.
    d. Severe dyskaryosis.

31. a. 股骨颈骨折。
   b. 骨质疏松症。
   c. 脊骨、桡骨和股骨颈。
   d. 长期的雌二醇缺乏，应用类固醇激素和甲状旁腺机能亢进。
   e. 显著的发病率，第一年的发病率 20%。

   a. Left fractured neck of femur.
   b. Osteoporosis.
   c. The spine, radius, neck of femur.
   d. Prolonged oestrogen deficiency, steroids, hyperparathyroidism.
   e. Significant morbidity and a 20% mortality in the first year.

32. a. 骨质疏松和脊椎压缩性骨折。
   b. 背痛、身高缩短；一些病例可无症状。
   c. 早绝经、白种的高加索人、家族史、既往长期闭经史和月经过少史。
   d. 小梁状的骨。
   e. 对外出感到恐慌且害怕再次骨折，抑郁，如果肋弓达到骨盆缘，会难以买到合适的衣服以及出现呼吸困难。

   a. Osteoporosis and vertebral crush fracture.
   b. Back pain, loss of height; in some cases no symptoms.
   c. Early menopause, white Caucasian, family history, past history of prolonged amenorrhoea or oligomenorrhoea.
   d. Trabecular bone.
   e. Anxiety about going out of doors and fear of further fractures, depression, difficulty in obtaining clothes to fit and respiratory problems if the rib cage rests on the pelvic brim.

33. a. 骨密度测定法。
   b. 35 岁左右（虽然还有些争议）。
   c. 充足的摄入钙剂和做一些承重的锻炼。
   d. 每年丢失少于 1%。
   e. 每年丢失 1% ~ 6% 或更多，通常是 2% ~ 3%。

   a. Bone densitometry.
   b. Mid-thirties (although this is somewhat contentious).
   c. Adequate calcium intake and weightbearing exercise.
   d. Less than 1% per year.
   e. 1%~6% per year or greater (typically 2%~3%).

34. a. 双能量X线吸收仪。
   b. 骨肿瘤。
   c. 单光子吸收测定法、双光子吸收测定法、定量的计算机体层扫描摄影、X线平片和超声检查。
   d. 沃式三角位于股骨颈，可用来测定绝经后的骨质丢失。
   e. 减少了检查时间，增加了精密度。

   a. Dual energy X-ray absorptiometry.
   b. Bone mass.
   c. Single photon absorptiometry, dual photon absorptiometry, quantitative computer tomography, plain X-ray and ultrasound.
   d. Ward's triangle is an area in the neck of femur that measures the earliest site of postmenopausal bone loss.
   e. Decreased scanning time, increased precision.

35. a. 正在植入性激素埋植片。
   b. 雌二醇和/或睾酮。
   c. 可作为一种性激素替代疗法。
   d. 可每6个月给药一次。
   e. 如果这个妇女有子宫应给予孕激素。

   a. Insertion of a hormone implant.
   b. Estradiol and/or testosterone.
   c. As a form of hormone replacement therapy.
   d. Every 6 months.
   e. If the woman has a uterus she should have progestogens.

36. a. 特纳综合征。
   b. 45，XO。
   c. 身材矮小、蹼颈、臂外斜角增大、性发育不成熟、原发性闭经和乳头发育不良。
   d. 不能。
   e. 超声检查（可看到水泡状淋巴管瘤）、绒毛膜绒毛取样、羊膜腔穿刺和脐带穿刺。

   a. Turner's syndrome.
   b. 45, X0.
   c. Short stature, webbed neck, increased carrying angle, sexual infantilism, primary amenorrhoea and widely spaced nipples.
   d. No.

e. Ultrasound scan (cystic hygroma), chorionic villus sampling, amniocentesis, cordocentesis.

37. a. 水肿的小囊泡。
b. 滋养细胞疾病。
c. 闭经伴阴道流血。妊娠反应重。
d. 典型的妊娠症状。子宫大小各异，但通常大于相应的月份，且无胎心。
e. 超声可确诊。吸出宫内容物并监测血HCG，在相关部门登记。建议避孕6个月至2年。

a. Hydropic vesicles.
b. Trophoblastic disease.
c. Amenorrhoea followed by vaginal bleeding. Exaggerated symptoms of pregnancy.
d. Typical signs of pregnancy. Uterine size variable but normally larger than dates. Absent fetal heart sounds.
e. Confirm diagnosis with ultrasound scan. Suction evacuation of uterus. Careful monitoring of HCG level. Registration with an appropriate centre. Advise avoidance of pregnancy for 6 months to 2 years.

38. a. 行宫腔镜检查。
b. 二氧化碳、甘氨酸或生理盐水。
c. 可直视下看到宫腔。切除内膜息肉或内膜切除术等操作过程也可通过宫腔镜进行。

a. Hysteroscopy.
b. CO_2, glycine or normal saline.
c. Visualize the endometrial cavity. Procedures can also be performed through the hysteroscope, e.g. removal of endometrial polyps or endometrial ablation.

39. a. 正进行静脉肾盂照影（intravenous pyelogram，IVP）。
b. 双侧的肾集合系统扩张。右侧的输尿管清晰可见直至骨盆缘。而左侧的输尿管仅中段可见。有外部肿物压迫膀胱。
c. 尿频、尿急和继发的肾感染症状。
d. 子宫肌瘤和卵巢肿瘤。

a. Intravenous pyelogram (IVP).
b. Bilateral dilatation of the pelvicalyceal system. The right ureter is

easily seen until the pelvic brim. Only the proximal portion of the left ureter can be seen. There is an extrinsic mass effect on the bladder.
c. Urinary urgency, frequency and symptoms secondary to renal tract infection.
d. Fibroid uterus, ovarian mass.

40. a. 醋酸。
b. 可见一个非常清晰的醋酸白区。
c. 轻微病变。
d. 非典型核细胞局限于上皮层三分之一。
e. 能。

a. Acetic acid.
b. There is a clearly defined area of aceto white.
c. Minor lesion.
d. Nuclear atypia confined to the basal third of the epithelium.
e. Yes.

41. a. 正常。
b. 禁性生活 3 天，将手淫获取的标本迅速送到实验室。
c. 在排卵期性交 6 小时内吸取宫颈黏液。
d. 阳性试验：在宫颈黏液中可见到活动的精子。这就排除了宫颈疾病导致的不孕，并且证实已发生了阴道性交。阴性试验可由除外宫颈黏液的其他多种因素导致，如不合适的时机或感染。

a. Normal.
b. 3 days abstinence from ejaculation, rapid transport to the laboratory of a specimen obtained by masturbation.
c. Aspiration of a sample of cervical mucus around the time of ovulation within 6 hours of intercourse.
d. Positive test: motile sperm in cervical mucus. This excludes cervical problem and confirms that vaginal intercourse has occurred. A negative test can be caused by many factors other than mucus hostility, for example poor timing or infection.

42. a. 既往月经规律而出现闭经 6 个月。
b. 下丘脑、垂体、内分泌（甲状腺、肾上腺）卵巢和生殖道。
c. 神经性厌食，主要是下丘脑受影响。
d. 血清泌乳素和卵泡刺激素水平。甲状腺机能测定。是否进一步检查由临床特征和一些基础检查的结果来决定。

a. Absence of periods for 6 months in a previously menstruating woman.
b. Hypothalamus, pituitary, endocrine (thyroid, adrenal), ovary, genital outflow tract.
c. Anorexia nervosa. Hypothalamus.
d. Serum prolactin and FSH levels. Thyroid function test. Further investigations are determined by the clinical features and results of the baseline tests.

43. a. 手术和放疗。
b. 病灶的大小和分期，同时考虑年龄、体重和患病妇女身体状况。
c. 可切除子宫、宫颈和一小部分阴道，同时包括子宫骶骨和主韧带。同时探查盆腔淋巴结。
d. *最上界*是髂外动脉。
*最下界*是输尿管。

a. Surgery and radiation therapy.
b. The size and stage of the lesion, together with the age, weight and general medical condition of the woman.
c. The uterus and cervix together with a cuff of vagina, the uterosacral and cardinal ligaments. In addition there is a pelvic node dissection.
d. *Uppermost tape*: external iliac artery.
Lowermost tape: ureter.

44. a. Ⅰ期和Ⅱa的宫颈癌妇女，无肥胖，年龄小于65岁且身体健康。
b. 髂总、髂外和髂内以及闭孔淋巴结。
c. *早期*: 流血、感染、瘘管形成、静脉血栓栓塞。
晚期: 膀胱机能障碍（张力减低）和淋巴囊肿形成。
d. 手术可保留卵巢和有功能的阴道。手术“一次”完成，使患者认为病灶已被“清除”。很少发生慢性膀胱和肠管的功能异常。而放疗适于疾病各期，绝大多数患者不会考虑她们的身体一般状况。卵巢功能无法保留，阴道也可能挛缩。大约8%的病人可发生远期膀胱和肠管的功能异常，多是由于放射线导致的纤维化而引起。

a. Carcinoma of the cervix stage I and stage IIa in a woman who is non-obese, usually less than 65 years of age, and otherwise in reasonable health.

b. The common iliac, external and internal iliac, and obturator lymph nodes.

c. *Early*: haemorrhage, infection, fistula, venous thromboembolism. *Late*: bladder dysfunction (hypotonia) and lymphocyst formation.

d. Surgery allows conservation of the ovaries and leaves a functional vagina. The treatment is completed 'at one sitting' and the woman knows that the cancer has been 'removed'. There are fewer chronic bladder and bowel disturbances. Radiation therapy can be used in all stages of disease and in the vast majority of patients irrespective of their general medical condition. Ovarian function will not be conserved and the vagina may become stenosed. Long-term bowel and bladder disturbance due to radiation fibrosis can be seen in up to 8% of patients.

45. a. 精子。
b. 分为头、颈和尾。
c. 曲细精管。
d. 卵泡刺激素。
e. 产生睾酮。

a. A spermatozoon.
b. Head, neck and tail.
c. Seminiferous tubules.
d. Follicle-stimulating hormone (FSH).
e. Production of testosterone.

46. a. 每年每 100 名妇女约 4 例。
b. 避孕套的乳头用前需挤压，在接触生殖道前，将避孕套套在勃起的阴茎上。射精后在阴茎未变软前即应按住套子的基底部将阴茎拔出。
c. 提供有效的避孕、易携带、容易使用、无须医学监督、防止性传播性疾病。
d. 给予事后避孕。

a. 4 per 100 woman years.
b. The teat needs to be squeezed, and the sheath unravelled over the erect penis prior to any genital contact. Following ejaculation the still erect penis needs to be withdrawn while holding on to the base of the condom.
c. Provides effective contraception, portable, easy to use, does not

require medical supervision and prevents sexually transmitted diseases.

d. Offer postcoital contraception.

47. a. 透热圈，可用来大范围环形切除移行带区。

b. 诊断和或治疗宫颈的癌前病变。

c. 应进行宫颈涂片和阴道镜检查。

d. 冷冻疗法、冷凝法、超短波电凝法、激光气化疗法、锥切和子宫切除术。

e. 出血、感染、宫颈狭窄。术后会有阴道排液，应指导患者避免使用阴道棉塞及性交。

a. The diathermy loop has been used to perform a large loop excision of the transformation zone.

b. Diagnosis and/or treatment of premalignant conditions of the cervix.

c. Cervical smear test, colposcopy.

d. Cryotherapy, cold coagulation, radical electrocoagulation diathermy, laser vaporization, cone biopsy (cold knife or laser), hysterectomy.

e. Haemorrhage, infection, cervical stenosis. A discharge occurs following the procedure and the patient should be advised to avoid the use of tampons and intercourse for the duration of the discharge.

48. a. 通常不确定，无特异症状，比较显著的是胃肠道的反应。压力增高的症状，如尿频同时伴有下腹的不适和腹胀可能存在。

b. 如恶病质、淋巴结病、胸腔积液、乳房病变、腹水、饼状大网膜和来自盆腔的肿物（？固定性）。

c. 全血细胞计数、生化检查、胸部X线、CA125水平和超声检查。有时也需要其他检查如钡剂灌肠和内镜检查。

d. 剖腹手术。

e. 卵巢上皮性肿瘤（极可能是恶性）。

a. Usually vague, non-specific symptoms, particularly of a gastrointestinal nature. Pressure symptoms such as urinary frequency may be present, together with lower abdominal discomfort and distention.

b. Signs of cachexia, lymphadenopathy, pleural effusions, breast pathology, ascites, omental cake lesion, mass arising from the pelvis (? fixity).

c. Full blood count, biochemical screen, chest X-ray, CA 125 level, ultrasound scan. Other tests sometimes required include barium enema and endoscopy.
d. At laparotomy.
e. Ovarian epithelial cell tumour (most probably malignant).

49. a. 尖锐湿疣。
b. 人乳头瘤病毒。
c. 是一种性传播疾病。
d. 期待治疗、鬼柏树脂（严密监测下使用）、冷灼术、电灼术、手术切除（很少用）、激光切除和干扰素。
e. 需告知病人该疾病具有性接触传播的特性，明显的病灶可被清除，而亚临床病灶无法治愈。而且可能复发。同时需检查性伴侣，与新的性伴侣进行性交需戴避孕套，而且要定期接受宫颈涂片检查。

a. Condylomata acuminata.
b. Human papilloma virus.
c. This is a sexually transmitted disease.
d. Expectant, podophyllin (with great care), cryocautery, electrocautery, excision (rarely), laser ablation and interferon.
e. The sexually transmissible nature of the condition needs to be discussed. Obvious lesions can be removed but subclinical disease cannot be cured. Recurrences are possible and the partner needs assessment. Condoms should be worn with any new sexual partners. Regular cervical cytology is important.

50. a. 卵巢癌。
b. 主要的播散方式是通过腹腔种植。也可通过淋巴和血液播散。
c. 大网膜是经常转移的部位，所以切除大网膜对确定分期十分重要，大网膜切除术可减少随后腹水的发生。
d. 主要的预测因素是病人的年龄和肿瘤的分期以及经彻底的开腹术后残留病灶的多少。

a. Ovarian carcinoma.
b. The main method of spread is via the peritoneal cavity. Lymphatic and haematogenous spread also occur.
c. The omentum is a frequent site of metastatic disease, so its removal is essential in staging the disease. Omentectomy may reduce subsequent incidence of ascites.

d. The main prognostic factors are the patient's age together with stage of the tumour and amount of residual disease at completion of laparotomy.

51. a. 宫颈前唇已被醋酸染白。可见镶嵌现象并伴随异常的血管。
b. CIN Ⅲ。
c. 可行阴道镜引导下的取点活检或环切。
d. 不能。

a. Areas on the anterior lip of the cervix have been stained white with acetic acid. Mosaicism is seen along with abnormal vessels.
b. CIN III.
c. Either a colposcopically directed punch biopsy or loop diathermy.
d. No.

52. a. 双侧乳头分泌乳样物。
b. 乳漏症（高泌乳素血症）。
c. 闭经和不孕。
d. 测定血清泌乳素水平，如升高，应通过 X 线、CT 或 MRI 来检查垂体窝。

a. Milky discharge from both nipples.
b. Galactorrhoea.
c. Amenorrhoea or infertility.
d. Serum prolactin level and if this is raised an X-ray, CT or MRI of the pituitary fossa.

53. a. CIN Ⅲ和浸润性鳞状细胞癌。
b. 如果是 I 期宫颈癌可行 Wertheim 子宫切除术。
c. 可以。

a. CIN III and invasive squamous cell carcinoma.
b. Assuming stage I carcinoma of the cervix, Wertheim's hysterectomy.
c. Yes.

54. a. 原发性梅毒性下疳。
b. 苍白螺旋体。
c. 潜伏期平均为 3 周，但也在 10 ~ 90 天。
d. 通过暗视野显微镜可看到螺旋体。
e. 确诊后，需向患者说明配合治疗和随访的必要性。需除外并发感染。可用青霉素治疗，禁性生活，追踪接触者。

a. Primary syphilitic chancre.
b. Treponema pallidum.
c. The incubation period averages 3 weeks but may range from 10-90 days.
d. Demonstration of spirochaetes by dark field microscopy.
e. Confirm the diagnosis and explain the need for compliance and follow-up. Exclude concurrent infections. Parenteral penicillin, abstinence from sex, contact tracing.

55. a. 输精管。
b. 输精管切除术。
c. 告知病人手术的性质、手术的效果、潜在的不可逆转性及极小的失败率。手术后患者在精液分析确定无精子之前一定不要认为已经绝育。
d. 阴囊血肿、慢性的阴囊不适、输精管自然吻合而导致节育失败，精囊的肉芽肿和抗精子抗体的产生。

a. Vas deferens.
b. Vasectomy.
c. The nature and effect of the operation together with the potential irreversibility and small failure rate. Postoperatively, the patient must not consider himself sterile until semen analyses confirm azoospermia.
d. Scrotal haematoma, chronic scrotal discomfort, spontaneous reanastomosis of the vas with consequent failure, spermatic granulomas and development of antisperm antibodies.

56. a. 内膜取样做组织学活检。
b. 无须麻醉。
c. 妊娠、慢性宫颈炎、最近或正患盆腔感染。
d. 放入阴道窥器，消毒宫颈，用单齿钳钳夹宫颈前唇，探测宫腔深度，并将取样器放入宫腔，扶稳取样器的套管，同时快速回拉取样器的活塞，取出取样器，并将组织置入适当的转移液中。
e. 子宫痉挛、子宫绞痛、子宫穿孔。

a. Endometrial sampling in order to obtain a histological biopsy.
b. Nil.
c. Pregnancy, chronic cervicitis, current or recent pelvic inflammatory disease.

d. Insert vaginal speculum and clean cervix, apply single toothed forceps to the anterior lip of the cervix, sound the uterus, insert the sampler into the uterine cavity, steady the sampler's sheath while rapidly pulling back the piston, withdraw the sampler and express the tissue into an appropriate transport medium.

e. Uterine spasm or cramping, perforation.

57. a. Filschie 绝育夹。

b. 使输卵管闭合。

c. 患者应了解此操作的含义，并且要提及其不可逆转性、失败率、并发症和风险，甚至可能需要行小切口开腹术。

d. 失败率是 2‰ ~ 3‰。

a. Filschie sterilization clip.

b. Tubal occlusion.

c. The patient must understand the implications of the procedure. You must discuss the potential irreversibility, the failure rate, the risks and complications of the procedure, and the small risk of a minilaparotomy being required.

d. 2~3 per 1000.

58. a. 子宫体。

b. 子宫骶骨韧带。

c. 不，少量游离的腹水通常可见。

d. 大肠。

a. Uterine body.

b. Uterosacral ligaments.

c. No, a small amount of free peritoneal fluid is commonly seen.

d. Large bowel.

59. a. 子宫输卵管造影片。

b. 检查不孕（子宫畸形、检测输卵管通畅性），输卵管手术后检测输卵管的通畅性，有时在困难的绝育术后证实输卵管是阻塞的。

c. 过敏反应、盆腔痛（输卵管痉挛）、盆腔炎复发。

d. 双角子宫且两侧可流出染色剂。

a. Hysterosalpingogram.

b. Investigation of infertility (uterine anomalies, check tubal patency), check on tubal patency after tubal surgery and occasionally verification of tubal occlusion after a difficult sterilization procedure.

c. Anaphylactic reaction, pelvic pain (tubal spasm), reactivation of pelvic infection.

d. Bicornuate uterus with bilateral free spill of dye.

60. a. 慢性外阴炎、全身瘙痒症、寄生虫感染、接触性皮炎、外阴上皮内瘤变、糖尿病、心理因素、念珠菌病和滴虫感染。

b. 综合临床表现，对局部治疗的反应 ± 活检。

c. 可局部应用高效价的类固醇激素，如无效需考虑活检。

a. A chronic vulval dermatosis, a generalized pruritic condition, parasitic infection, contact dermatitis, VIN, glycosuria, psychological causes, candidiasis and trichomoniasis.

b. A combination of clinical appearance, response to topical treatments ± biopsy.

c. Topical high potency steroids. If no response consider biopsy.

61. a. 腹腔镜下染色剂灌注。

b. 检测不孕，在输卵管手术后检测输卵管的通畅性。

c. *腹腔镜检查*: 全身麻醉下可对盆腔器官进行全面检查，并可检查输卵管的通畅性，内膜异位病灶和输卵管周围的粘连灶也可看到。

子宫输卵管造影术: 可在门诊进行，检测子宫和输卵管。但由于输卵管痉挛，导致较高的假阴性率。无法反映盆腔的情况。受检妇女的卵巢会接受一定量的放射线辐射。

d. 正常的输卵管，有明显的染色剂流出。

a. Laparoscopy with dye instillation.

b. Investigation of infertility, check on tubal patency after tubal surgery.

c. *Laparoscopy*: general anaesthetic but allows full inspection of the pelvic organs and check on tubal patency.
Endometriosis and fine peritubal adhesions also seen.
Hysterosalpingography: outpatient procedure that outlines the uterus and internal tubal structure, but the false negative rate, due to tubal spasm, is higher. No information regarding the peritoneal cavity. The ovaries of the woman receive a dose of irradiation.

d. Normal fimbrial ends with obvious spill of dye.

62. a. 先兆流产。

b. 不可避免流产。

c. 完全性流产。
d. 不完全性流产。
e. 稽留流产。

a. Threatened.
b. Inevitable.
c. Complete (expelled products).
d. Incomplete.
e. Delayed.

63. a. 在左侧外阴的后外侧可见高尔夫球大小的肿物，未合并感染。
b. 巴氏腺囊肿。
c. 由于腺管的扩张而不是由于腺体本身的原因。
d. 如果合并感染会导致巴氏腺脓肿。
e. 囊肿造口术是最简单的治疗方案。

a. Golf-ball-sized swelling in the left posterolateral vulva. No associated inflammation.
b. Bartholin's cyst.
c. These cysts result from dilatation of the duct rather than of the gland itself.
d. If infection occurs a Bartholin's abscess will result.
e. Marsupialization of the cyst is the simplest treatment.

64. a. 子宫内膜癌。
b. 未产妇、肥胖、高血压、糖尿病和无对抗的雌激素治疗。
c. 宫腔镜检查、内膜活检或正规的宫颈扩张和诊刮术。
d. 腺癌。
e. 直接蔓延到邻近组织、淋巴和血液播散，脱落细胞从输卵管溢出。
f. 经腹全子宫切除术和双侧附件切除术，手术分期 ± 辅助性放疗。

a. Endometrial carcinoma.
b. Nulliparity, obesity, hypertension, diabetes mellitus and unopposed oestrogen therapy.
c. Hysteroscopy and endometrial biopsy or formal dilatation and curettage.
d. Adenocarcinoma.
e. Direct spread to adjacent structures, lymphatic and haematogenous spread and spillage of exfoliated cells from the tubes.

f. Total abdominal hysterectomy and bilateral salpingooophorectomy, surgical staging ± adjuvant radiation therapy.

65. a. 经腹全子宫切除术。
b. 没有。
c. 阴道。
d. 可吸收线来缝合。

a. Total abdominal hysterectomy.
b. No.
c. The vagina.
d. An absorbable polyfilament suture e.g. vicryl.

66. 1= 左侧卵巢纤维瘤。
2= 子宫。
3= 右输卵管。
4= 术者的手指。
5= 膀胱。
6= 大肠。

1 = left ovarian fibroma.
2 = uterus.
3 = right fallopian tube.
4 = surgeon's finger.
5 = bladder.
6 = large bowel.

67. a. 细菌性阴道病。
b. 可见明显的线索细胞。
c. 线索细胞由上皮细胞和大量粘附的细菌组成，特征的致病菌是阴道加尔纳菌。
d. 灰色、稀薄、均质、有异味的分泌物。
e. 甲硝唑 400mg 口服，一日两次，共服 5 日。

a. Bacterial vaginosis.
b. A clue cell is evident.
c. The clue cell is an epithelial cell with numerous adherent bacteria. The characteristic organism is Gardnerella vaginalis.
d. Thin, grey, homogeneous, odorous discharge.
e. Metronidazole 400mg orally twice a day for 5 days.

68. a. Fitz-Hugh-Curtis 综合征。
    b. 肝周炎。
    c. 沙眼衣原体。
    d. 出现盆腔感染和不孕的症状和体征。
    e. 四环素（也可土霉素 100mg 一日两次）共 14 天，性伴侣也需治疗。

    a. Fitz-Hugh-Curtis syndrome.
    b. Perihepatitis.
    c. Chlamydia trachomatis.
    d. Signs and symptoms of pelvic infection and infertility.
    e. Tetracycline (e.g. doxycycline 100mg twice daily) for 14 days and ensure partner is treated.

69. a. 阴道前壁。
    b. 膀胱。
    c. 感到盆腔压力，感觉有东西要掉下来，不能排空膀胱，如存在膀胱颈的旋转性下降会出现压力性尿失禁。
    d. 阴道前壁修补术。
    e. 会出现尿道肉阜。

    a. Anterior vaginal wall.
    b. Bladder.
    c. Pelvic pressure, a feeling of something coming down, incomplete bladder emptying. Urinary stress incontinence may be present if there is rotational descent of the bladder neck.
    d. Anterior colporrhaphy.
    e. Urethral caruncle.

70. a. 双侧输卵管积水且无染色剂流入腹腔。
    b. 盆腔炎。
    c. 输卵管伞端。
    d. 输卵管手术（腹腔镜或开腹手术）或体外受精。

    a. Bilateral hydrosalpinges with no spill of dye into the peritoneal cavity.
    b. Pelvic inflammatory disease.
    c. The terminal aspect of the fallopian tubes.
    d. Tubal surgery (laparoscopic or open laparotomy) and in-vitro fertilization.

71. a. 阴式子宫切除术。
b. 子宫骶韧带和主韧带。当子宫与阴道呈90° 角时，圆韧带和阔韧带也起到支撑作用。
c. 膀胱、直肠、尿道、输尿管和小肠。
d. 出血、感染、血栓性疾病、损伤周围组织的并发症、肠梗阻、盆腔血肿。

a. Vaginal hysterectomy.
b. Uterosacral and cardinal ligaments. Other support is provided by the uterus lying at 90° to the vaginal axis and the round and broad ligaments.
c. Bladder, rectum, urethra, ureter and small bowel.
d. Haemorrhage, infection, thromboembolic disease, sequelae of damage to surrounding structures (e.g. fistula), ileus, pelvic haematoma.

72. a. 宫颈息肉。
b. 绝经后出血。
c. 间质可有扩张的宫颈内隐窝。表皮组织通常是柱状上皮且能分泌黏液，也可表现为鳞状上皮化生。
d. 息肉切除术、宫腔镜检查以及宫颈扩张和刮宫术。
e. 在门诊行拧除术。

a. Cervical polyp.
b. Postmenopausal bleeding.
c. There is a stroma that contains dilated endocervical crypts. The surface epithelium is usually columnar and mucus-secreting. The surface epithelium may show squamous metaplasia.
d. Polypectomy, hysteroscopy and dilatation and curettage.
e. Twist avulsion as an outpatient procedure.

73. a. 可用来避孕。
b. 雌二醇和孕激素。
c. ①调控月经周期。
②减少流血。
③减轻腹痛。
④减少卵巢癌的发生。
⑤减少子宫内膜癌的发生。
⑥减缓骨量丢失。

⑦减轻内膜异位症的症状。

⑧改善痤疮症状。

⑨减少盆腔炎的发生。

d. 无需任何处置。

e. 活动性血栓栓塞性疾病，雌激素依赖性肿瘤。

a. Contraception.

b. Oestrogen and Progestogen.

c. ① Cycle control.

② Less bleeding.

③ Less pain.

④ Protects against ovarian cancer.

⑤ Protects against endometrial cancer.

⑥ Prevents bone loss.

⑦ Alleviates symptoms of endometriosis.

⑧ Acne Improvement.

⑨ Protects against PID.

d. Nothing.

e. Active thromboembolic disease, oestrogen dependent tumours.

74. a. A. 卵泡刺激素。

B. 黄体生成素。

C. 雌二醇。

D. 孕激素。

b. 卵泡膜细胞和颗粒细胞。

c. 黄体内黄素化的颗粒细胞。

d. 它使黏液变得黏稠不利于精子穿透。

e. 孕激素。

f. 2 百万（1 百万至 4 百万）。

a. A. FSH.

B. LH.

C. Estradiol.

D. Progesterone.

b. Theca cells of the stroma and granulosa cells of the follicle.

c. Luteinised granulosa cells of the corpus luteum.

d. It makes mucus hostile or impenetrable to sperm.

e. Progesterone.

f. 2 million (1-4 million).

75. a. 性交后出血和月经间期出血。

b. 立即行阴道镜检查并请妇科专家行活组织检查。

c. 行 Wertheim 子宫切除术或放疗。

d. ①多个性伴侣。

② HPV16 和 HPV18 感染。

③吸烟。

④既往有宫颈上皮内瘤样病变（CIN）。

⑤有性传播性疾病病史（STD）。

⑥过早性生活。

e. 80%。

f. 50 ~ 60 岁。

a. Postcoital bleeding and intermenstrual bleeding.

b. Refer immediately for colposcopy and refer to gynaecologist for biopsy.

c. Wertheim's hysterectomy or radiotherapy.

d. 1. Large number of sexual partners.

2. HPV 16 and 18.

3. Smoking.

4. Previous cervical intraepithelial neoplasia (CIN).

5. History of sexually transmitted disease (STD).

6. Early age of first coitus.

e. 80%.

f. 50~60 years.

76. a. 不自主排尿，导致一系列社会和个人卫生问题。

b. 膀胱逼尿肌出现了问题。

c. ①压力性尿失禁 / 负荷性尿失禁。

②尿频 / 尿急 / 排尿困难。

③夜尿症 / 遗尿症。

d. ①膀胱训练 / 膀胱锻炼。

②减少进水量，尤其在夜间更应如此。

e. 抗胆碱能药物。

f. 普鲁本辛水胶物 15mg，一日两次。

a. This is a condition in which there is involuntary loss of urine, leading to a social or personal problem with hygiene.

b. Detrusor instability.

c. ① Stress incontinence/urge incontinence.

② Frequency/urgency/dysuria.
③ Nocturia/enuresis.
d. ① Bladder drill/bladder training.
② Reduction in fluid intake, especially in the evening.
e. Anticholinergic drugs.
f. Propanthelinehydrocloride 15 mg B.D.

77. a. 性激素替代疗法。
b. ①雌激素依赖的肿瘤 / 乳腺癌 / 子宫内膜癌。
②活动性肝病 / 慢性活动型肝炎 / 急性肝炎。
c. ①防止骨质疏松 / 骨质丢失 / 保持骨质。
②防止结肠直肠癌。
d. 经皮肤的孕激素和含孕激素的宫内节育器。
e. 尽管予以高水平的药物或雌激素仍会出现一定的症状。
f. 在给药之前应测定血清雌二醇水平，严格按照时间植入（例如间隔时间不少于 6 个月）。

a. Hormone replacement therapy.
b. ① Oestrogen-dependent tumour/breast carcinoma/endometrial carcinoma.
② Active liver disease/chronic active hepatitis/acute hepatitis.
c. ① Prevention of osteoporosis/bone loss/preservation of bone.
② Prevention of colorectal cancer.
d. Transdermal progestogen and intrauterine progestogen-containing device.
e. Return of symptoms despite high levels of drug/oestrogen.
f. Measure serum estradiol prior to administration. Strict adherence to time of giving implants (i.e. not less than 6 months apart).

78. a. 子宫纤维瘤。
b. ①腹胀。
②不孕。
③排尿困难。
④腹痛。
⑤经量增多。
c. 出血和损伤其他器官如输尿管、膀胱和肠管。
d. 可能需要输血和或子宫切除术。
e. ①胎方位异常。
②尿潴留。

③胎盘早剥 / 产前出血。

f. 0.2%。

a. Fibroid uterus.

b. ① Abdominal distension.
② Infertility.
③ Difficulty with micturition.
④ Abdominal pain.
⑤ Menorrhagia.

c. Haemorrhage and damage to other organs, e.g. ureter, bladder, bowel.

d. A blood transfusion and/or hysterectomy may be needed.

e. ① Abnormal lie.
② Urinary retention.
③ Placental abruption/APH.

f. 0.2%

79. a. 膀胱减压测定法和尿流量测定 / 尿动力学测定。

b. > 15ml/s。

c. 真性压力性尿失禁。

d. ①减轻体重。
②戒烟。
③治疗便秘。
④盆底肌练习。
⑤物理疗法。
⑥感应电疗法。
⑦阴道锥。

e. ①阴式手术：例如阴道前壁修补 /Pacey/Kelly 修补术。
②经腹手术: Burch阴道悬吊术/Marshall-Marchetti-Krantz术。
③阴腹联合手术：Stamey 手术。

f. 阴道悬吊术。

g. 80% ~ 90%。

a. Subtraction cystometry and uroflowmetry/urodynamic studies.

b. > 15 ml/s.

c. Genuine stress incontinence.

d. ① Weight loss.
② Stop smoking.
③ Treat constipation.
④ Pelvic floor exercises.

⑤ Physiotherapy.
⑥ Faradism.
⑦ Vaginal cones.
e. ① Vaginal approach, e.g. anterior colporraphy/Pacey/Kelly repair.
② Abdominal approach, e.g. Burch colposuspension/ Marshall-Marchetti-Krantz.
③ Combined abdominovaginal approach, e.g. Stamey procedure.
f. Colposuspension.
g. 80%~90%.

80. a. 宫腔镜检查。
b. 子宫内膜息肉。
c. 切除息肉。
d. 1. 宫颈息肉 / 宫颈畸形 / 宫颈癌。
2. 子宫内膜增生。
3. 子宫内膜癌。
4. 激素治疗。
5. 黏膜下肌瘤。
e. ①生理盐水。
②甘氨酸。
③二氧化碳。
f. 良性。
g. 经阴式扫描。

a. Hysteroscopy.
b. Endometrial polyp.
c. Removal of the polyp.
d. ① Cervical polyp/cervical abnormality/cervical carcinoma.
② Endometrial hyperplasia.
③ Endometrial carcinoma.
④ Hormone therapy.
⑤ Submucous fibroid.
e. ① Normal saline.
② Glycine.
③ CO_2.
f. Benign.
g. Transvaginal scan.

81. a. 阴道镜检查，可看到正常宫颈。
b. 生理盐水、醋酸和卢戈碘。

c. 异型细胞，这是细胞学诊断。

d. 这是一个组织学概念，它描述了上皮层的部分组织由不同程度的核异型细胞取代的这样一种病变。

a. A colposcope. It shows a normal cervix.

b. Normal saline, acetic acid and Lugol's iodine.

c. Abnormal cells. This is a cytological diagnosis.

d. This is a histological term and describes a lesion in which part of the thickness of the epithelium is replaced by cells showing varying degrees of nuclear atypia.

专业词汇英中对照

A

abdominal mass	腹部肿块
abortion, see miscarriage; therapeutic abortion	流产，流产；治疗性流产
absent vagina	无阴道
acetowhite'reaction,	醋酸白实验
mosaicism	镶嵌现象
acyclovir	阿昔洛伟
adenocarcinoma	腺癌
endometrial	子宫内膜的
ovarian	卵巢的
adhesions	粘连
endometriosis	子宫内膜异位症
pelvic	骨盆的
perihepatitis	肝周炎
AIDS indicator diseases	艾滋病标志性疾病
5α reductase deficiency	5α 还原酶缺乏
ambiguous genitalia	两性生殖器
amenorrhoea	闭经
galactorrhoea	溢乳
in polycysitic ovary symdrome	多囊卵巢综合征
primary	原发性
secondary	继发性
anal trauma	直肠损伤
androgen production ovarian	产生雄激素，卵巢肿瘤
anorexia nervosa	神经性厌食
anovulatory dysfunctional bleeding	无排卵性功血
anterior colporrhaphy	阴道前壁修补术
antiphospholipid antibody syndrome	抗磷脂抗体综合征
antisperm antibodies	抗精子抗体
asherman's syndrome	艾什曼综合征
Aylesbury spatula	Aylesbury 刮勺

B

bacterial vaginosis	细菌性阴道病
bartholin's cyst /abscess	巴氏腺囊肿或脓肿
bartholin's glands	巴氏腺
basal body temperature chart	基础体温表
benign cystic teratoma (dermoid cyst)	良性囊性畸胎瘤（皮样囊肿）
beta-HCG	β -HCG
bicornuate uterus	双角子宫
bilateral salpingo-oophorectomy and total abdominal hysterectomy	腹式全子宫、双侧附件切除术
bimanual examination	双合诊
biopsy	活组织检查
colposcopically directed cone	阴道镜下的宫颈锥切
follow-up	随访
endometrial	子宫内膜的
bivalve speculum	双瓣窥器
bladder drill	膀胱训练
bleeding	出血
dysfunctional uterine	功能失调性的子宫
intraperitoneal	腹膜内的
bone densitometry	骨密度测定
botryoid sarcoma	葡萄状肉瘤
bowel herniation	肠疝
bruising in sexual abuse	性虐待擦伤

C

CA 125	CA 125
cancer, *see specific conditions*	癌症，见特殊疾病
candida infections /candidiasis	念珠菌感染 / 念珠菌病
in AIDS	艾滋病
caps	帽
carbon dioxide inflation of abdomen	腹腔内二氧化碳充气
carcinoma, *see specific carcinomas*	癌，见特殊癌
cervical carcinoma	宫颈癌
cervical smear	宫颈涂片
histology	组织学

invasive	浸润的
management	处理
premalignant /microinvasive disease	恶变前 / 微小浸润疾病
radiotherapy	放疗
staging	疾病分期
cervical excitation	宫颈刺激症
cervical intraepithelial neoplasia	宫颈上皮内瘤变（CIN）
CIN Ⅰ	CIN Ⅰ
CIN Ⅲ	CIN Ⅲ
cervical mucus	宫颈黏液
cervical smear	宫颈涂片
results from	起因于
cervicitis	宫颈炎
cervix	宫颈
double	两个
normal	正常的
child sex abuse	儿童性虐待
childhood disorders	儿童期疾病
congenital	先天性的
early childhood	幼童期
chlamydio trachomatis	沙眼衣原体
‘chocolate cysts’	“巧克力囊肿”
choriocarcioma	恶性蜕膜瘤
climacteric	更年期的
clindamycin	克林霉素
clomiphene	克罗米酚
clotrimazole	克霉唑
clue cell	线索细胞
colour doppler ultrasonography	彩色多普勒超声检查法
ovarian blood flow	卵巢血流
colporrhaphy, anterior	阴道缝合术，前壁
colposcopy	阴道镜检查
cervix	宫颈
mosaicism of	镶嵌现象
normal	正常的
colposuspension	阴道悬吊术
columnar epithelium	柱状上皮

combined oral contraceptive pills	复合型口服避孕药
complete hydatidiform mole	完全性葡萄胎
complete miscarriage	完全流产
expelled products	排出物
condoms	避孕套
condylomata acuminate	尖锐湿疣
cone biopsy	锥切活检
follow-up	随访
contraception	避孕
barrier methods	屏障法
and HIV	和人类免疫缺陷病毒
hormonal	激素法
natural	自然法
postcoital	性交后的
cornual blockage	角部闭锁
corpus luteum	黄体
counseling	咨询
after condylomata acuminate	患尖锐湿疣后
infertility	不孕症
therapeutic abortion	治疗性流产
cuscoe's speculum	cuscoe 窥器
cystocele	膀胱膨出
cystometry	膀胱测压
subtraction	减压

D

danazol	达那唑
delayed miscarriage	稽留流产
ultrasonography	超声波检查
depot progestogen injections	己酸羟孕酮注射
dermoid cyst (being cystic teratoma)	皮样囊肿（囊性畸胎瘤）
detrusor instability	逼肌功能失调
diagnosis	诊断
diaphragms	膈
diathermy loop	透热圈
diathermy loop excision	电热环切术
dilation and evacuation	宫颈扩张术和宫腔吸刮术

disseminated ovarian adenocarcinoma 播散性卵巢腺癌
distension cysts 扩张囊
dorsal position 仰卧位
dowager's hump 贵妇式驼背
dual energy x-ray absorptiometry 双能量X线吸光测定
dyskaryotic cells 核异质细胞
  colposcopy 阴道镜检查
  histology 组织学检查
dysplasia 发育异常

E

econazole 益康唑
ectocervix 子宫颈阴道部
ectopic pregnancy 异位妊娠
  diagnosis 诊断
  fetus in peritoneal cavity 腹腔妊娠
  management 处理
  ultrasomography 超声波检查
embryological abnormalities 胚胎发育异常
embryonal rhabdosarcoma 胚胎横纹肌肉瘤
endocervial canal 宫颈管
endocervical swabs 宫颈内拭子
endometrial cancer 子宫内膜癌
  radiotherapy 放射疗法
endometrial lining removal 内膜线去除
endometrial sampling 子宫内膜标本
endometriomas 子宫腺肌瘤
endometriosis 子宫内膜异位症
  cervical 宫颈的
  and infertility 和不孕症
  laparoscopic surgery 腹腔镜手术
  laparoscopic view 腹腔镜检查
  management 处理
endometriotic deposit 子宫内膜异位灶
endometrium 子宫内膜
  biopsy 活组织检查
  changes in menstrual cycle 在月经周期中的变化

examination	检查
dysfunctional bleeding	功能失调性出血
enterocele	肠疝
epidermoid cyst	皮样囊肿
episiotomy, anterior	外阴侧切术，前面的
epithelial ovarian tumours	卵巢上皮性肿瘤
estradiol	雌二醇
implants in HRT	在性激素替代治疗埋植剂中
in menstrual cycle	在月经周期中
evacuation of uterus	子宫的排出物
examination	检查
instruments	器械
positions	体位
techniques	技术
bimanual examination	双合诊检查
cervical smear	宫颈涂片
colposcopy	阴道镜检查
hysterosalpingo contrast	子宫输卵管对比造影
sonography	超声检查
hysterosalpingography	子宫输卵管造影
hysteroscopy	宫腔镜检查
laparoscopy	腹腔镜检查
swabs, microbiological	拭子，微生物学的

F

fallopian tubes	输卵管
benign /malignant conditions	良/恶性疾病
blockage testing, see tubal patency testing	阻塞试验，见输卵管通畅性检查
cancer	癌症
ectopic pregnancy	异位妊娠
laparoscopic view	腹腔镜下探查
normal	正常的
female genital mutilation	女性生殖器缺如
ferryman and Gallway scoring system	Ferryman 和 Gallway 评分系统
fibroids	纤维瘤
cervical	宫颈的
endometrial	子宫内膜的

uterine	子宫的
fibroma, ovarian	纤维瘤，卵巢的
Filschie sterilization clip	Filschie 节育夹
fistulous track	瘘管
Fitz-Hugh-Curtis syndrome	Fitz-Hugh-Curtis 综合征
fluconazole	氟康唑
follicle monitoring	卵泡监测
follicle-stimulating hormone	卵泡雌激素
in menopause /climacteric	在绝经期 / 更年期中
in menstrual cycle	在月经周期中
follicular cysts	滤泡囊肿
Fothergill repair	Fothergill 修补术
fractured neck of femur	股骨颈骨折
FSH, see follicle-stimulating hormone	卵泡刺激素
Fused labia	阴唇粘连

G

galactorrhoea	溢乳
gamete intrafallopian transfer	输卵管内配子移植术
gemeprost	吉美前列素
genital mutilation	生殖器缺如
germ-cell-derived ovarian tumours	生殖细胞来源的卵巢肿瘤
gestrinone	内美通
gonadotrophins	促性腺激素
in infertility	在不孕症中
in menstrual cycle	在月经周期中
in polycystic ovary syndrome	多囊卵巢综合征
gonadotrophin-releasing hormone	促性腺激素释放激素
gonadotrophin-relaeasing hormone analogues	促性腺激素释放激素类似物

H

haematocolpos	阴道积血
HCG, see human chorionic gonadotrophin	人绒毛膜促性腺激素
herpes genitalis	生殖器疱疹
herpes simplex virus (HSV)	单纯疱疹病毒
high vaginal swabs	阴道上部涂片

hirsutism	多毛症
history taking	病史采集
form	形式
infertility	不育史
HIV infection	人类免疫缺陷病毒感染
Hodge pessaries	Hodge 子宫托
hormonal changes in menstrual cycle	在月经周期中激素的变化
hormone implants	激素埋植剂
contraception	避孕
replacement therapy	替代疗法
hormone replacement therapy	性激素替代疗法
implants	埋植剂
hyman chorionic gonadotrophin (HCG)	人绒毛膜促性腺激素
in ectopic pregnancy	在异位妊娠中
in menstrual cycle	在月经周期中
human immunodeficiency virus (HIV)	人免疫缺陷病毒
human papilloma virus (HPV)	人乳头状瘤病毒
and cervical carcinoma	和宫颈癌
and VIN/CIN	和 VIN/CIN
hydatidiform mole	葡萄胎
ultrasonography	超声波检查
hydrocolpos	阴道积液
hydropic vesicles	水肿囊泡
hydrosalpinges	输卵管积水
bilateral	双侧
hyperprolactinaemia	高泌乳素血症
hyperstimulation in polycystic ovaries	多囊卵巢的过度刺激症
hypogonadotropnic hypogonadism	低促性腺激素性腺机能减退
hypothalamic-pituitary-ovarian axis	下丘脑 - 垂体 - 卵巢轴
hypothalamic suppression	下丘脑抑制
hysterectomy	子宫切除术
in cervical carcinoma	在宫颈癌中
total abdominal	经腹全子宫
and bilateral salpingo-oophorectomy	和双侧附件切除术
vaginal	阴道的
wertheim's	wertheim 术
hysterosalpingo contrast sonography (HyCoSy)	子宫输卵管对比造影声像图检查

hysterosalpingography (HSG)	子宫输卵管造影术
fallopian tubes	输卵管
tubal infection	输卵管感染
tubal patency	输卵管通水
hydrosalpinges	输卵管积水
uterus	子宫
bicornuate	双角的
vs laparoscopy	*vs* 经腹腔镜检查
hysteroscopy	宫腔镜检查
endometrial	子宫内膜的
endometrial cancer	子宫内膜癌
endometrial polyps	子宫内膜息肉

I

in vitro fertilization (IVF)	体外受精
incomplete miscarriage	不全流产
incontinence, see urinary incontinence	失禁，见尿失禁
inevitable miscarriage	难免流产
infections	感染
genital mutilation	生殖器缺如
gynaecological	妇科的
record keeping	文件保存
tubal	输卵管的
see also specific infections	见特殊感染
infertility	不孕症
and endometriosis	和子宫内膜异位症
examination	检查
female	女性
galactorrhoea	溢乳
male	男性
and pelvic inflammatory disease	和盆腔炎
in polycystic ovary syndrome	在多囊性卵巢综合征中
unexplained	无法解释的
intersex	雌雄间体
intracytoplasmic sperm injection (ICSI)	卵浆内单精子注射
intratubal /intraperitoneal bleeding	输卵管或腹腔内出血
intrauterine contraceptive devices (IUCDs)	宫内节育器

and pelvic inflammatory disease	和盆腔炎
intrauterine system, progesterone-releasing (IUS)	宫内系统，释放孕酮
intravenous pyelogram(IVP)	肾盂静脉造影
invasive hydatidiform mole	侵袭性葡萄胎

K

Kaposi's sarcoma	卡波西肉瘤
Krukenberg tumours	Krukenberg 瘤

L

labioplasty	阴唇成形术
laparoscopy	腹腔镜检查
bicornuate uterus	双角子宫
colposuspension	阴道悬吊术
dye instillation for tubal patency	输卵管通畅的染色剂注入
endometriosis	子宫内膜异位症
fallopian tubes	输卵管
pelvic adhesions	盆腔粘连
laser cautery	激光烧灼器
levonorgestrdl	左旋 -18- 甲基炔诺孕酮
leydig cells	睾丸间质细胞
lH see luteinizing hormone	促黄体生成素
lichen sclerosus	硬化性苔藓
Lloyd-Davies position	Lloyd-Davies 体位
luteinizing hormone	促黄体生成素
in menstrual cycle	在月经周期中
in polycystic ovary syndrome	在多囊性卵巢综合征中
lymph node removal	淋巴结摘除术
uterine cancer	子宫癌
Wertheim's hysterectomy	Wertheim 子宫切除术

M

Manchester repair	Manchester 修补术
medroxyprogesterone acetate	醋酸甲羟孕酮
menopause	绝经期
bone loss	骨丢失

menstrual cycle	月经周期
see also amenorrhoea ;oligomenorrhoea	也见闭经；月经过少
metaplasia of coelomic epithelium	体腔上皮化生
metronidazole	甲硝唑
micturating cystogram	膀胱X线照片
mifepristone	米非司酮
miscarriage	流产
causes	病因
recurrent	复发
types	类型
mosaicism of cervix	宫颈的镶嵌现象
mucus hostility	黏液黏稠
Mullerian ducts	苗勒管

N

neisseria gonorrhoea	淋病

O

obstructed labour	分娩梗阻
oestrogen	雌二醇
in contraception	在避孕中
and fused labia	和阴唇融合
in hormone replacement therapy	在激素代替疗法中
in menopause /climacteric	在绝经期/更年期中
in menstrual cycle	在月经周期中
oligoamenrrhoea	月经过少
omentectomy	网膜切除术
oocyte aspiration	卵母细胞抽吸术
oral contraceptive pills	口服避孕药
for endometriosis	用于子宫内膜异位症
for polycystic ovary syndrome	用于多囊性卵巢综合征
postcoital	性交后的
osteoporosis	骨质疏松症
osteoporotic wedge fractures	骨质疏松引起的楔状骨折
ovarian blood flow	卵巢血流量
ovarian cancer	卵巢癌
abdominal distension	腹胀

ovarian cysts, physiological distension	卵巢囊肿，生理性扩张
ovarian fibroma	卵巢纤维瘤
ovarian hyperstimulation	卵巢过度刺激症
ovarian mass	卵巢肿物
ovarian tumours	卵巢肿瘤
benign	良性
derivation	诱因
ovaries	卵巢
overflow incontinence	溢流性尿失禁
ovulatory dysfunctional bleeding	有排卵的功能失调性出血

P

Paget's disease of vulva	外阴 Paget 病
partial hydatidiform mole	部分性葡萄胎
pelvic examination positions	经骨盆检查胎位
pelvic inflammatory disease	盆腔炎
and intrauterine contraceptive devices (IUCDs)	和宫内节育器
perihepatitis	肝周炎
pessaries for prolapse	子宫托
pituitary fossa, enlarged	垂体窝，扩大
pneumocystis carinii	卡氏肺囊虫
polycystic ovaries	多囊卵巢
kissing	相吻合
ultrasonography	超声波检查
polycystic ovary syndrome (PCOS)	多囊性卵巢综合征
polyps	息肉
cervical	宫颈的
endometrial	子宫内膜的
pedunculated	带蒂的
postcoital test	性交后试验
postmenopausal bleeding	绝经后阴道流血
pouch of douglas in ectopic pregnancy	异位妊娠时的直肠子宫陷凹
powder burns	热灼伤
pregnancy	妊娠
detection	检测
early problems	早期问题

premalignent conditions	癌前病变
cervical	宫颈的
vulval intraepithelial neoplasia	外阴上皮内瘤变
see also cervical intraepithelial neoplasia	也见宫颈上皮内瘤变
procidentia	脱垂
in vaginal hysterectomy	经阴道子宫切除术
progesterone	黄体酮
implants	埋植剂
in menstrual cycle	在月经周期中
progesterone antagonists	黄体酮拮抗剂
progesterone-only pill	黄体酮——仅有片剂
progesterone releasing intrauterine system(IUS)	孕激素宫内释放系统
progestogens	孕激素
in contraceptive pill	在避孕药中
in hormone replacement therapy	在激素代替疗法中
injections in contraception	在避孕药针剂中
propantheline hydrochloride	盐酸普鲁本辛
prostaglandins	前列腺素
pruritus vulvae	外阴瘙痒
puberty	青春期
disorders of	紊乱
punctuation of cervix	宫颈标记

R

radiotherapy	放射疗法
cervical carcinoma	宫颈癌
endometrial cancer	子宫内膜癌
uterine cancer	子宫癌
rectocele	直肠膨出
recurrent miscarriage	习惯性流产
5α reductase deficiency	5α 还原酶缺乏
retrograde menstruation	经血逆流
rhabdosarcoma, embryonal	横纹肌肉瘤，胚胎期的
rhythm method of contraception	安全期避孕法
ring pessaries	环形子宫托

S

salpingectomhy	输卵管切除术
see and treat system	访问和治疗体系
semen analysis, normal	精液分析，正常的
Semm cautery	Semm 烧灼
serous tumours	浆液性瘤
Sertoli-Leydig tumours	Sertoli-Leydig 细胞瘤
sex abuse, child	性虐待，儿童
sheehan syndrome	席汉综合征
shelf pessaries	架型子宫托
Sims position	西姆斯体位
Sims speculum	西姆斯窥器
smoking	吸烟
and cervical carcinoma	和宫颈癌
and uterovaginal prolapse	和子宫阴道脱垂
specula	窥器
bivalve	双瓣
Cuscoe's	Cuscoe
Sims	西姆斯
spermatozoon	精子
spermicidal sponges	杀精子棉球
squamocolumnar junction	鳞状 - 柱状上皮交界处
staging	分期
cervical cancer	宫颈癌
ovarian cancer	卵巢癌
uterine cancer	子宫癌
sterilization	绝育术
sterilization clip	节育夹
strawberry cervix	草莓状宫颈
stress incontinence	压力性尿失禁
stromal ovarian tumours	卵巢间质瘤
subtraction cystometry	膀胱减压测定法
swabs, microbiological	拭子，微生物学的
sexual abuse	性滥交
syphilis	梅毒
syphilitic chancre	梅毒硬下疳

T

tachyphylaxis	快速免疫法
temperature	体温
and contraception	和避孕
in infertility	和不孕症
tension-free vaginal tape (TVT) procedure	无张力阴道悬吊术
teratoma, benign cystic (dermord cyst)	畸胎瘤，良性囊性的（皮样囊肿）
testicular feminization	睾丸女性化
testosterone implants in HRT	在激素替代疗法中的睾酮埋植剂
tetracycline	四环素
therapeutic abortion	治疗性流产
forms	形式
threatened miscarriage	先兆流产
thrush	鹅口疮
total abdominal hysterectomy	经腹全子宫切除术
and bilateral salpingo- oophorectomy	和双附件切除术
toxoplasmosis of brain	脑弓形虫病
trachelectomy, radical	宫颈切除术，根本的
transformation zone	移行带
large loop excision	较大的环形切除术
treponema pallidum	苍白密螺旋体
trichomonas vaginalis	滴虫性阴道炎
trophoblastic disease	滋养细胞疾病
tubal disorders	输卵管疾病
abscesses(hydrosalpinges)	脓肿（输卵管积水）
infection	感染
occlusion	阻塞
rupture	破裂
tubal patency testing	输卵管通畅试验
tubo-ovarian abscesses, bilateral	输卵管卵巢脓肿，双侧
Turner's symdrome	特纳综合征

U

ultrasonography	超声波检查
delayed miscarriage	稽留流产
ectopic pregnancy	异位妊娠
endometrial	子宫内膜的

follicle monitoring	卵泡监测
hydatidiform mole	葡萄胎
polycystic ovaries	多囊卵巢
urethral caruncle	尿道肉阜
urethral diverticulum	尿道憩室
urethrocele	尿道膨出
urinary incontinency	尿失禁
overflow	反流性
stress	压力性
true	真性
urge	加负荷
urodynamic investigations	尿动力学研究
uterine bleeding, dysfunctional	功能失调性子宫出血
uterine body	子宫体
uterine cancer	子宫癌
uterine cavity	子宫腔
uterine prolapse	子宫脱垂
uterosacral ligaments	子宫骶骨韧带
uterovaginal prolapse	子宫阴道脱垂
management	处理
uterus	子宫
bicornuate	双角的
congenital anomalies	先天畸形
evacuation of	排泄物
retroverted	后倾的

V

vagina	阴道
absent	缺如
cytology showing oestrogenic stimulation	细胞学检查显示雌激素刺激
vaginal bruising	阴道裂伤
vaginal carcinoma	阴道癌
vaginal cones	阴道锥
vaginal septum	阴道隔
vaginal swabs	阴道拭子
vaginal wall pressure necrosis	阴道壁压迫性坏死
vaginal wall prolapse	阴道壁膨出

vaginitis	阴道炎
vaginosis, bacterial	阴道病，细菌性
vas deferens	输精管
vasectomy	输精管切除术
vertebral crush fracture	脊椎压缩性骨折
videocystourethrography	可视膀胱尿道造影术
virilism	男性化
vulval bruising	外阴裂伤
vulval carcinoma	外阴癌
invasive	浸润性
vulval dermatoses	外阴皮肤病
vulval epithelial disorders	外阴上皮内的病变
vulval intraepithelial neoplasia	外阴上皮内瘤变
vulvovaginitis	外阴阴道炎

W

Ward's triangle	沃氏三角
wart virus, see human papilloma virus	疣病毒，见人乳头状瘤病毒
warts	疣
cervical	宫颈的
vulval /vaginal	外阴的 / 阴道的
wedge fractures of spine	脊柱楔形骨折
Wertheim's hysterectomy	Wertheim 子宫切除术